MW01195235

Simplified Regenerative Procedures for Intraosseous Defects

SIMPLIFIED REGENERATIVE PROCEDURES
for Intraosseous Defects

Edited by

Leonardo Trombelli, DDS, PhD

Full Professor and Chair, Periodontology

Director, Research Centre for the Study of Periodontal
and Peri-Implant Diseases
University of Ferrara

Operative Unit of Dentistry
Azienda Unità Sanitaria Locale di Ferrara
Ferrara, Italy

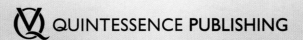

QUINTESSENCE PUBLISHING

Berlin | Chicago | Tokyo
Barcelona | London | Milan | Mexico City | Moscow | Paris | Prague | Seoul | Warsaw
Beijing | Istanbul | Sao Paulo | Zagreb

To my mentor, Prof Giorgio Calura, with gratitude

Library of Congress Cataloging-in-Publication Data

Names: Trombelli, Leonardo, editor.

Title: Simplified regenerative procedures for intraosseous defects / edited by Leonardo Trombelli.

Description: Chicago : Quintessence Publishing Co, Inc, [2020] | Includes bibliographical references and index. | Summary: "Atlas presenting surgical and nonsurgical methods to treat intraosseous defects, with a focus on the single-flap approach, including indications and contraindications for treating defects with each method and detailed descriptions of the steps required for each procedure"-- Provided by publisher.

Identifiers: LCCN 2019047285 (print) | LCCN 2019047286 (ebook) | ISBN 9780867159455 (paperback) | ISBN 9780867159929 (ebook)

Subjects: MESH: Periodontal Diseases--surgery | Guided Tissue Regeneration, Periodontal--methods | Surgical Flaps | Atlas

Classification: LCC RK361.A1 (print) | LCC RK361.A1 (ebook) | NLM WU 17 | DDC 617.6/32059--dc23

LC record available at https://lccn.loc.gov/2019047285

LC ebook record available at https://lccn.loc.gov/2019047286

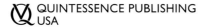

QUINTESSENCE PUBLISHING
USA

© 2020 Quintessence Publishing Co, Inc

Quintessence Publishing Co, Inc
411 N Raddant Road
Batavia, IL 60510
www.quintpub.com

5   4   3   2   1

Editor: Marieke Zaffron
Design: Sue Zubek
Production: Angelina Schmelter

Printed in the USA

CONTENTS

Video content

 Extra video content is available online wherever indicated by a QR code. Scan the QR code here or in the text to access this supplementary information. The full list of videos may also be found at www.quintpub.com/Trombelli/Simplified-Regenerative-Procedures_Videos.

FOREWORD

It is always a great satisfaction when you are asked to write a foreword of a good book. This is especially true when the book expands our scientific culture and promotes the training of our students and professionals. Frequently, these books introduce new knowledge or new technologies. However, it is less frequent for a book to be purposely focused on training students and professionals on surgical procedures. This atlas focuses on evidence-based education and in acquiring relevant professional competencies in the surgical treatment of specific periodontal lesions (ie, intraosseous defects). The information provided is clear, well organized, and very practical, but at the same time it is rigorous and up to date with current knowledge, comprehensively covering the fundamentals of periodontal regeneration and the use of the different technologies. It particularly focuses on simplified surgical procedures aimed to attain the best possible regenerative outcomes with minimal invasiveness.

The author, Prof Leonardo Trombelli, has dedicated many years of his professional life to studying and researching successful long-term periodontal therapy and specifically the use of regenerative surgical interventions to improve the prognosis of periodontally affected teeth. He has published essential scientific articles that provide the basis for this book. His contribution to this work clearly demonstrates not only his excellent scientific background but also the teaching abilities that are needed to produce a book such as this, with scientific rigor and at the same time with practical relevance for students and professionals. Moreover, the many contributors in this work are not only well respected in Italy but also in Europe and beyond.

In summary, this book is clear and well written and provides very useful and relevant content to support dentists and periodontists in learning how to apply modern periodontal surgical interventions to achieve regeneration in teeth that have lost periodontal attachment as a consequence of periodontitis.

Mariano Sanz, MD, DDS, Dr Med
Professor and Chairman, Periodontology
Faculty of Odontology
Complutense University of Madrid
Madrid, Spain

PREFACE

Man should be as eager to simplify his life as he is to complicate it.
—Henri-Louis Bergson

For 20 years, in collaboration with the whole research group at the Research Centre for the Study of Periodontal and Peri-Implant Diseases, University of Ferrara, we have been making a great effort in trying to find diagnostic and therapeutic solutions that could optimize endpoints while making clinical processes and pathways easier for practitioners and students. We started back in 2007 with a simplified method to access deep intraosseous defects (the *single-flap approach*, or SFA, that will be extensively described in this book). Then, in 2008, we introduced the Smart Lift technique—a simplified, standardized method to perform sinus elevations with a minimally invasive transcrestal surgical procedure (a method that has been extensively investigated and published on for more than 10 years). In 2009, we reported on a simplified method to assess the periodontal risk profile of the patient, based on five straightforward parameters that have been shown to be linked to the progression of periodontal breakdown. And more recently, in 2018, we published on a simplified method for horizontal bone augmentation, which is based on the creation of a periosteal pouch that acts as an osteogenic, space-providing membrane for bone grafting (the subperiosteal peri-implant augmented layer, or SPAL technique).

The development of simplified procedures has been a main focus of my career for two main reasons. First, I want to provide the profession with simple, straightforward, innovative solutions that may bring clinicians closer to procedures that are otherwise neglected because of their potential complexity. In search of simplified diagnostic and treatment procedures, we targeted those that are mostly perceived as successful only when performed by the talented and gifted hands of a few select colleagues. I am well aware that spreading the use of simplified procedures among dental professionals means amplifying the number of patients who may benefit from them. The second reason is related to my mission as a university faculty member. Teaching simple procedures can help the great majority of students to reach a high level of competence in a reasonable amount of time with a fast learning curve.

These two reasons represent the main driving force that brought me to write this book. With the large number of photographs and videos of many different clinical cases, the textbook has been designed as a sort of tutorial for both graduate students and practitioners who want to expand their knowledge and technical skill in the nonsurgical and surgical treatment of deep intraosseous defects, very common lesions in patients with Stage III and IV periodontitis. In particular, the SFA is thoroughly described with a step-by-step approach, starting from the analysis of diagnostic and prognostic patient/defect characteristics to the selection of surgical instruments, choice of flap design, methods for root debridement and conditioning, use of appropriate regenerative technologies, description of suitable suture techniques for different flap designs, and the short- and long-term postsurgery care. A multitude of clinical cases are illustrated in great detail in order to provide a wide range of scenarios and conditions where the SFA can be easily and successfully applied.

In conclusion, I wish to acknowledge all the coauthors who have contributed to make this textbook a unique, up-to-date manual on regenerative procedures: Anton Sculean, Dieter Bosshardt, and Raluca Cosgarea, who have thoroughly described the fundamental principles of periodontal regeneration; Mario Aimetti, Giulia Mariani, and Federica Romano, who described novel nonsurgical approaches; and Roberto Farina for his talented help with the surgical chapter. A special thanks to Anna Simonelli, who spent a great amount of her postgraduate education and PhD program coordinating and monitoring a massive amount of clinical research on the SFA. Without her precious work, this textbook would have never reached such a level of quality and completeness. Also, I want to express my sincere gratitude to Quintessence Publishing, who from the very first moment has strongly and convincingly believed in this challenging editorial project. Last but not least, I want to thank my family: my wife, Cristina, and my children Emma and Andrea for their continuous, silent, and patient support.

CONTRIBUTORS

Mario Aimetti, MD, DDS
Associate Professor, Periodontology
Department of Surgical Sciences
Dental School
University of Turin
Turin, Italy

Dieter D. Bosshardt, PhD
Associate Professor
Department of Oral Surgery and Stomatology
School of Dental Medicine
University of Bern
Bern, Switzerland

Raluca Cosgarea, DDS
Assistant Professor
Department of Periodontology
Philipps University of Marburg
Marburg, Germany

Assistant Professor
Department of Prosthetic Dentistry
Iuliu Hațieganu University of Medicine
   and Pharmacy
Cluj-Napoca, Romania

Roberto Farina, DDS, PhD, MSc
Associate Professor, Oral Surgery
Research Centre for the Study of
   Periodontal and Peri-Implant Diseases
University of Ferrara

Operative Unit of Dentistry
Azienda Unità Sanitaria Locale di Ferrara
Ferrara, Italy

Giulia Maria Mariani, DDS, MSc
Visiting Professor, Periodontology
Department of Surgical Sciences
Dental School
University of Turin
Turin, Italy

Federica Romano, DDS
Research ssistant, Periodontology
Department of Surgical Sciences
Dental School
University of Turin
Turin, Italy

Anton Sculean, DMD, Dr hc, MSc
Full Professor and Chair, Periodontology
Department of Periodontology
School of Dental Medicine
University of Bern
Bern, Switzerland

Anna Simonelli, DDS, PhD
Research Fellow, Periodontology
Research Centre for the Study of
   Periodontal and Peri-Implant Diseases
University of Ferrara
Ferrara, Italy

Leonardo Trombelli, DDS, PhD
Full professor and Chair, Periodontology
Director, Research Centre for the Study of
   Periodontal and Peri-Implant Diseases
University of Ferrara

Operative Unit of Dentistry
Azienda Unità Sanitaria Locale di Ferrara
Ferrara, Italy

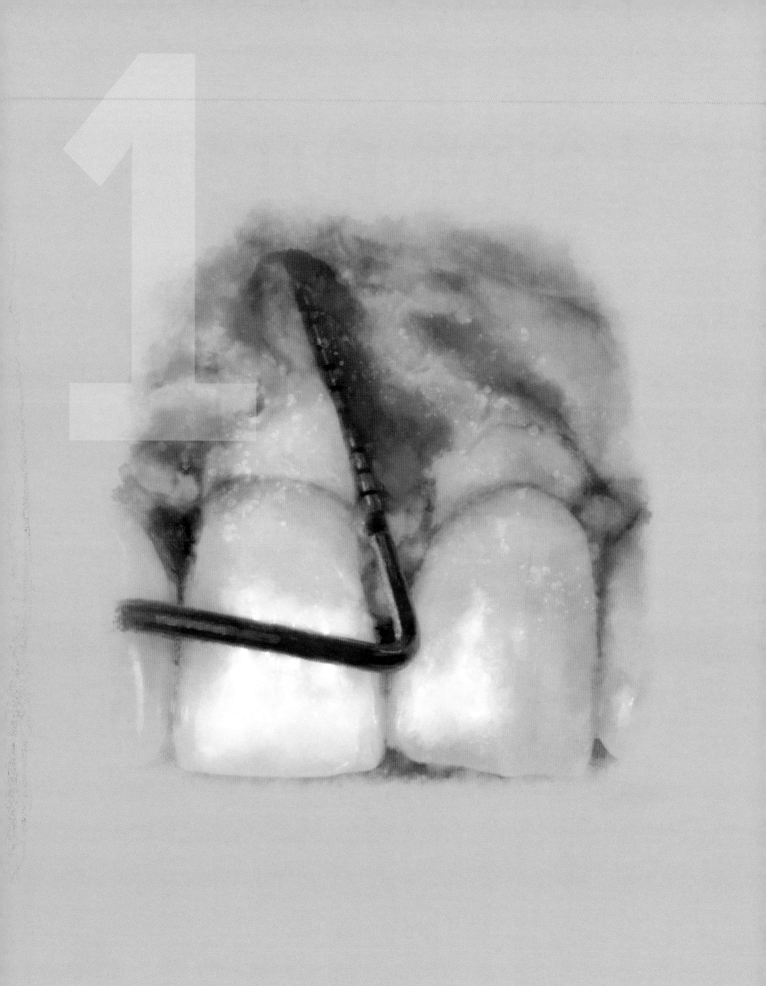

INTRODUCTION

Leonardo Trombelli, DDS, PhD
Roberto Farina, DDS, PhD, MSc
Anna Simonelli, DDS, PhD

WHY A TEXTBOOK ON THE TREATMENT OF INTRAOSSEOUS DEFECTS?

The prevalence of intraosseous defects in adults was investigated on dried skulls[1] as well as through clinical[2,3] and radiographic assessments.[4–8] At the patient level, the presence of at least one intraosseous defect was detected with an incidence ranging between 25.5% and 51% in samples representative of the general population or specific age cohorts,[1,6,7] between 18% and 23% in patients seeking dental care,[4,8] and of 45.1% in a periodontally compromised cohort.[2] A retrospective study revealed that intraosseous lesions are at high risk of further progression, and they may lead to tooth loss if left untreated.[9] Papapanou and Wennström[9] retrospectively recorded the bone level changes as well as tooth loss over a 10-year period at tooth sites with intraosseous defects in individuals not treated with systematic periodontal therapy. The results demonstrated an increased frequency of tooth loss and bone loss with increasing depth of the intraosseous defect. In particular, the proportion of teeth lost between the 1- and 10-year examinations was 22%, 46%, and 68% for teeth with a defect depth of 2 mm, 2.5 to 4 mm, and ≥ 4.5 mm, respectively.

These observations reinforce the need for:

- A proper diagnosis of the intraosseous defect, which represents a common lesion in patients affected by Stage III and IV periodontitis.
- An appropriate treatment of the lesion that may successfully revert those conditions (probing depth [PD] ≥ 5 mm associated with bleeding on probing [BOP]) conducive to progressive attachment/bone loss.

WHY A TEXTBOOK ON REGENERATIVE PROCEDURES?

The ideal outcome of the surgical treatment of a deep intraosseous defect is the regeneration of the tooth attachment apparatus destroyed by the process of periodontitis. From a histologic point of view, periodontal regeneration implies the formation of periodontal ligament fibers inserted into newly formed cementum and bone.[10] Data from human histologic studies have provided evidence that periodontal regeneration may be accomplished by using different regenerative technologies, including membranes and biologic agents[11–15] (see chapter 2).

Extensive clinical data have shown that compared with nonregenerative treatment, the surgical regenerative treatment of deep intraosseous lesions may result in a considerable improvement of probing parameters following the tissue maturation phase.[16–21] From a clinical point of view, periodontal regeneration may result in a substantial increase in clinical attachment level (CAL) gain (of at least 3 mm) and relevant bone fill of the intraosseous component of the lesion together with a maintainable, stable probing depth (ie, PD ≤ 4 mm in absence of BOP).

Sculean et al[22] published the results of a 10-year follow-up after the regenerative treatment of 38 intraosseous periodontal defects with different regenerative treatments: enamel matrix derivative (EMD), guided tissue regeneration (GTR), combination EMD and GTR, and open flap debridement (OFD). After treatment, all patients were placed in a 3-month supportive periodontal care program. At 1 year, a significantly greater CAL gain was achieved in the regeneration groups (ie, GTR, EMD, or combination) compared to OFD controls, and this was maintained substantially unvaried for a 10-year period.

A 20-year follow-up after regenerative treatment of intraosseous defects was recently reported in a cohort of 45 patients.[23] Defects were treated with three different modalities: GTR with modified papilla preservation flap, GTR with conventional access flap, and access flap alone without membrane. All patients were enrolled in a supportive periodontal care program with 3-month recalls. At both 1-year and 20-year reevaluation, a significantly better CAL gain and PD reduction was obtained by the two GTR treatments than the access flap. Moreover, the access flap surgery was associated with a greater disease recurrence.[23]

Collectively, available data seem to support the use of regenerative devices to ensure better short- and long-term outcomes than mere surgical debridement at deep intraosseous defects.

WHY A TEXTBOOK ON SIMPLIFIED TREATMENT PROCEDURES?

Despite decades of well-established nonsurgical and surgical protocols and techniques, the treatment of deep intraosseous lesions still represents a challenge for clinicians. There is a perception that the regenerative treatment of an intraosseous lesion is both technically sensitive and costly, with limited outcome predictability in the hands of the average operator (ie, not specially trained or highly skilled). This perception is likely due to aspects related to debridement of any lesions via a "closed" approach (see chapter 3) and those associated with the difficulty in performing a correct flap design and suturing technique as well as in selecting the appropriate regenerative technology. The purpose of this textbook is to present simplified procedures that may overcome these issues, at least in part, when treating an intraosseous defect.

The term *simplify* means the act of making something less complex. In the present textbook, we define a procedure aimed at improving the clinical conditions of a deep intraosseous lesion (in terms of substantial clinical and histologic attachment gain and bone fill, reduction of the PD to a maintainable condition, and limited to no postsurgery recession) as *simplified* when characterized by more favorable conditions for the patient and/or the clinical operator. Although the terms *simplification* and *minimal invasiveness* may appear as synonyms when referring to periodontal treatment, in our perspective *simplification* implies a substantially broader concept.

For the operator, a simplified procedure has the following characteristics[24]:

* Limited surgical equipment
* An easy-to-learn technique
* Limited need for additional treatments or devices (through the maximization of the inherent healing potential of the treated lesion)

For the patient, a simplified procedure should have a reduced impact on the following[24]:

* Posttreatment daily activities
* Posttreatment pain and discomfort (also reducing the required compliance for post-treatment regimens)
* Preexisting esthetics

For both patient and operator, a simplified procedure should reduce both treatment costs and chairside time needed for both treatment administration and follow up visits.[24] This also results in fewer treatment costs.

Nonsurgical therapy as a standalone treatment always represents a "simplified" procedure, particularly when compared with surgical approaches. Among the available surgical options, simplified surgical procedures share a common technical aspect (ie, the elevation of a single flap on the buccal or palatal/lingual aspect), leaving the tissues on the opposite side intact. In this respect, this textbook will focus in detail on a novel surgical approach—the single-flap approach—that was first introduced in 2007[25] and repeatedly validated by different randomized clinical trials thereafter (see chapter 4). The single-flap approach was shown to be at least as effective as traditional papilla preservation techniques when evaluated either as a standalone protocol or in combination with regenerative devices.

The main goal of this textbook is to show the effectiveness of simplified surgical procedures to treat challenging intraosseous lesions. The authors' ambition is to teach how clinicians may achieve substantial treatment outcomes associated with minimal esthetic impairment and a more tolerable postoperative course.

Simplifying both the nonsurgical and surgical treatment phases will achieve the following outcomes:

* Reshape the learning curve, thus increasing the generalizability of treatment outcomes
* Improve patient access to care by limiting biologic and economic costs

REFERENCES

1. Larato DC. Intrabony defects in the dry human skull. J Periodontol 1970;41:496–498.
2. Söder B, Jin LJ, Söder PO, Wikner S. Clinical characteristics of destructive periodontitis in a risk group of Swedish urban adults. Swed Dent J 1995;19:9–15.
3. Vrotsos JA, Parashis AO, Theofanatos GD, Smulow JB. Prevalence and distribution of bone defects in moderate and advanced adult periodontitis. J Clin Periodontol 1999;26:44–48.
4. Nielsen IM, Glavind L, Karring T. Interproximal periodontal intrabony defects. Prevalence, localization and etiological factors. J Clin Periodontol 1980:7:187–198.
5. Papapanou PN, Wennström JL, Gröndahl K. Periodontal status in relation to age and tooth type. A cross-sectional radiographic study. J Clin Periodontol 1988;15:469–478.
6. Wouters FR, Salonen LE, Helldén LB, Frithiof L. Prevalence of interproximal periodontal intrabony defects in an adult population in Sweden. A radiographic study. J Clin Periodontol 1989;16:144–149.
7. Soikkonen K, Wolf J, Närhi T, Ainamo A. Radiographic periodontal findings in an elderly Finnish population. J Clin Periodontol 1998;25:439–445.
8. Dundar N, Ilgenli T, Kal BI, Boyacioglu H. The frequency of periodontal infrabony defects on panoramic radiographs of an adult population seeking dental care. Community Dent Health 2008;25:226–230.
9. Papapanou PN, Wennström JL. The angular bony defect as indicator of further alveolar bone loss. J Clin Periodontol 1991;18:317–322.
10. Sander L, Karring T. Healing of periodontal lesions in monkeys following the guided tissue regeneration procedure. A histological study. J Clin Periodontol 1995;22:332–337.
11. Nyman S, Lindhe J, Karring T, Rylander H. New attachment following surgical treatment of human periodontal disease. J Clin Periodontol 1982;9:290–296.
12. Heijl L, Heden G, Svärdström G, Ostgren A. Enamel matrix derivative (EMDOGAIN) in the treatment of intrabony periodontal defects. J Clin Periodontol 1997;24:705–714.
13. Bosshardt DD, Sculean A, Windisch P, Pjetursson BE, Lang NP. Effects of enamel matrix proteins on tissue formation along the roots of human teeth. J Periodontal Res 2005;40:158–167.

14. Majzoub Z, Bobbo M, Atiyeh F, Cordioli G. Two patterns of histologic healing in an intrabony defect following treatment with enamel matrix derivative: A human case report. Int J Periodontics Restorative Dent 2005;25:283–294.

15. Nevins M, Kao RT, McGuire MK, et al. Platelet-derived growth factor promotes periodontal regeneration regeneration in localized osseous defects: 36-month extension results from a randomized, controlled, double-masked clinical trial. J Periodontol 2013;84:456–464.

16. Trombelli L, Heitz-Mayfield LJ, Needleman I, Moles D, Scabbia A. A systematic review of graft materials and biological agents for periodontal intraosseous defects. J Clin Periodontol 2002;29(suppl 3):117–135.

17. Giannobile WV, Somerman MJ. Growth and amelogenin-like factors in periodontal wound healing. A systematic review. Ann Periodontol 2003;8:193–204.

18. Trombelli L, Farina R. Clinical outcomes with bioactive agents alone or in combination with grafting or guided tissue regeneration. J Clin Periodontol 2008;35(suppl 8):117–135.

19. Koop R, Merheb J, Quirynen M. Periodontal regeneration with enamel matrix derivative in reconstructive periodontal therapy: A systematic review. J Periodontol 2012;83:707–720.

20. Matarasso M, Iorio-Siciliano V, Blasi A, Ramaglia L, Salvi GE, Sculean A. Enamel matrix derivative and bone grafts for periodontal regeneration of intrabony defects. A systematic review and meta-analysis. Clin Oral Investig 2015;19:1581–1593.

21. Kao RT, Nares S, Reynolds MA. Periodontal regeneration—Intrabony defects: A systematic review from the AAP Regeneration Workshop. J Periodontol 2015;86(suppl 2):S77–S104.

22. Sculean A, Kiss A, Miliauskaite A, Schwarz F, Arweiler NB, Hannig M. Ten-year results following treatment of intra-bony defects with enamel matrix proteins and guided tissue regeneration. J Clin Periodontol 2008;35:817–824.

23. Cortellini P, Buti J, Pini Prato G, Tonetti MS. Periodontal regeneration compared with access flap surgery in human intra-bony defects 20-year follow-up of a randomized clinical trial: Tooth retention, periodontitis recurrence and costs. J Clin Periodontol 2017;44:58–66.

24. Trombelli L, Simonelli A, Minenna L, Vecchiatini R, Farina R. Simplified procedures to treat periodontal intraosseous defects in esthetic areas. Periodontol 2000 2018;77:93–110.

25. Trombelli L, Farina R, Franceschetti G. Single flap approach in periodontal surgery [in Italian]. Dent Cadmos 2007;75:15–25.

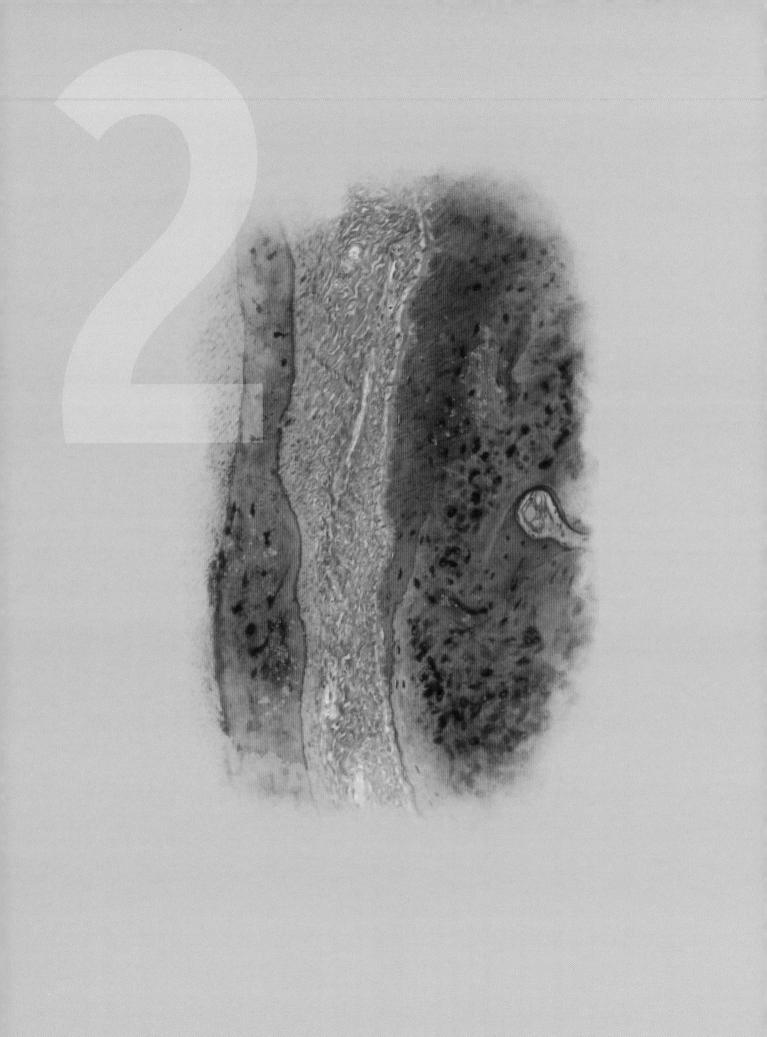

FUNDAMENTALS IN PERIODONTAL REGENERATION

Raluca Cosgarea, DDS

Dieter D. Bosshardt, PhD

Leonardo Trombelli, DDS, PhD

Anton Sculean, DMD, Dr hc, MSc

PRINCIPLES OF PERIODONTAL WOUND HEALING

Based on histologic observations, the healing process of a mucogingival flap at a tooth surface resembles that of epidermal wound healing.[1] This is characterized by an initial adhesion/adsorption of a fibrin clot to the wound margins, followed by early and late phases of inflammation, then formation of granulation tissue and a matrix. The final step of wound healing is tissue remodeling[2,3] (Fig 2 1). As opposed to epidermal wound healing (ie, epidermal incisions or excisions) where the opposing wound margins are two vascular gingival/mucosal margins, periodontal wound healing is different because healing occurs between a vascular surface (ie, epithelium, connective tissue) and an avascular, rigid, mineralized surface (ie, cementum or dentin). Additionally, tissue resources for the healing process derive from the mucogingival flap, the alveolar bone, and the periodontal ligament (PDL).

The periodontal healing process is initiated by adsorption/adhesion of plasma proteins (ie, blood-derived proteins) onto the exposed root surface at the time of flap closure, resulting in clot formation at the tooth-mucogingival interface.[4] This clot has a dual role as protection for the denuded tissues and as a provisional matrix for the consequent cell migration.[2] In the early phase of inflammation, which follows within hours after incision, inflammatory cells (ie, neutrophils and monocytes) colonize onto the root surface, cleansing the wound area from necrotic debris and bacteria via phagocytosis, enzymes, and toxic oxygen products. A few days later, macrophages invade the wound, and the late phase of inflammation begins. Macrophages sustain the release of various growth factors and cytokines, which in turn stimulate migration of various cells from the circumscribing tissues (fibroblasts, endothelial cells, etc), forming a cell-rich granulation tissue. This undergoes maturation and remodeling: fibroblasts replace the initial provisional matrix with a new matrix rich in collagen, and a connective tissue attachment is established by day 7. However,

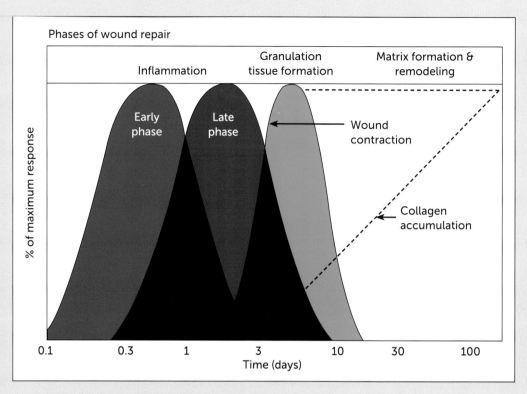

Fig 2-1 Phases of epidermal incisional wound healing, including an early (ie, within hours) and a late (ie, within days) phase of inflammation dominated by polymorphonuclear neutrophils and macrophages, respectively. The magnitude of wound contraction parallels the phase of granulation tissue formation. Collagen accumulation is first observed during the phase of granulation tissue formation, continuing through the phase of matrix formation and remodeling (courtesy of Dr Richard AF Clark).

depending on the wound size and the cell resources of the surrounding area, a fibrin clot may still be observed at the maturation stage. These observations underline the importance of allowing adhesion/adsorption of plasma proteins onto the root surface undisturbed to form new connective tissue attachment/periodontal regeneration.[1,4]

Epithelial versus connective tissue attachment

The type of healing—regeneration or repair/scar formation—is determined by the maturation of the granulation tissue in the periodontal wound.[5] This depends on the available cell types and signals that stimulate the migration of these cells into the granulation tissue.[5]

Healing in the form of periodontal repair is characterized by a long junctional epithelium (ie, epithelial attachment) between the mucogingival flap and the tooth surface (Fig 2-2). Additionally, a fibrous encapsulation (ie, collagen adhesion) may sometimes be observed with collagen fibrils coming in close vicinity to the root surface and forming a physicochemical attachment.[6] In other situations, the exposed root surface may present repair cementum (intrinsic fiber cementum), and parts of the exposed tooth structure may be replaced with connective tissue initiating root resorption or may be replaced by bone

Fig 2-2 Micrographs at low *(a)* and high *(b)* magnifications illustrating the formation of a long junctional epithelium (LJE), when no periodontal regenerative therapy was applied. The *arrowhead* marks the apical end of the junctional epithelium. B, bone; D, dentin; GM, gingival margin; OC, old cementum; P, dental pulp; PL, periodontal ligament.

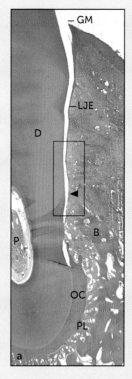
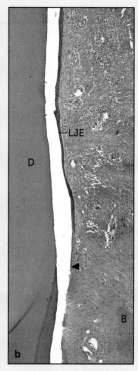

resulting in ankylosis.[7] Nonetheless, when newly formed collagen fibers are functionally oriented in newly formed cementum (cellular/acellular mixed/extrinsic fiber cementum), healing results in periodontal regeneration.

Early histologic studies pointed out the importance of an adhering fibrin clot to the root surface and its subsequent maturation to prevent an epithelial downgrowth and promote a connective tissue attachment.[8,9] In this sense, histologic experiments in critical-size defects in dogs (5-mm supra-alveolar periodontal defects) showed that an initial contamination of the root surface with heparin rather inhibits the formation/adhesion/adsorption of a fibrin clot and leads to healing with a long junctional epithelium.[10] Nonetheless, it was observed in further animal studies that wound-stabilizing measures like the use of a macropouros polylactic acid (PLA) matrix or an occlusive expanded polytetrafluoroethylene (ePTFE) barrier membrane to divert wound-rupturing forces inhibited the downgrowth of epithelial cells and sustained the maturation of the fibrin clot into a viable connective tissue attachment.[11,12] Thus, the formation, adhesion, and adsorption of a fibrin clot and its integrity against physiologic and/or wound-rupturing forces are critical for its maturation into connective tissue and therefore play a key role in periodontal healing via connective tissue attachment.[8,11,12] In the early healing phase, wound stability is assured by the passive adaptation of the flap and by suturing. Strategically placed holding and closing sutures have to overcome wound-rupturing tensile forces to ensure primary intention healing until wound maturation (14 days as shown in animal experiments for limited periodontal dehiscence defects).[8] Early suture removal or other traumatic postsurgical procedures (eg, mechanical tooth brushing, periodontal dressings) may interfere with the structural integrity of the wound.[1]

In 1976, Melcher was the first to hypothesize that the cells that initially adhere to the root surface determine the type of the new attachment.[13] In histologic studies, Karring et al not only confirmed this theory but also showed that the PDL has an enormous regenerative potential and further that it is the only structure with the capacity to regenerate the lost periodontal attachment.[14] When cells originating from the PDL are the first to repopulate the previously contaminated root surface, periodontal regeneration seems to occur predictably.[15–17] These research findings therefore suggested that using a barrier to block migration of cells originating from the mucogingival flap may allow the regeneration of lost periodontal tissues; thus, the concept of guided tissue regeneration (GTR) was born.

In this context, further histologic animal experiments evaluated the regenerative potential of PDL in various settings using the critical-size supra-alveolar periodontal defect model and different types of ePTFE membranes.[11,18–20] When the defects treated with ePTFE membranes were evaluated after 4 weeks of healing, bone regeneration was only detectable at sites where the membrane provided space. At 4 weeks of healing, neither cementum nor functionally oriented periodontal attachment could be observed. Moreover, at the sites where the membrane collapsed or wound failure occurred (eg, membrane exposure, infection, necrosis), no regeneration of any tissue could be observed.[11] However, in a subsequent study with a space-providing ePTFE membrane and an 8-week healing period, regeneration of all periodontal tissues (ie, alveolar bone, cementum, and functionally oriented PDL fibers) was noted on the entire exposed root surface. Limited regeneration of periodontal tissues was also observed in cases with membrane collapse or at control sites (no membrane), but inflammation and necrosis occurred at sites with membrane exposure.[18] Thus, it seems crucial to ensure wound healing by primary intention and space provision for a healing and regeneration period of at least 8 weeks to regenerate the lost periodontium.

Another histologic study in dogs treated surgically created periodontal defects with a space-providing nonobstructive gold mesh and showed that osteogenesis occurred even when occlusion of the gingival tissue was not assured.[21] A study testing a structurally reinforced space-providing macroporous ePTFE membrane and a semi-occlusive ePTFE membrane was performed in critical-size supra-alveolar periodontal defects, resulting in comparable significant regeneration of cementum, alveolar bone, and a functionally oriented PDL for both membrane types.[19] Nonetheless, 50% of the sites treated with the occlusive membrane experienced membrane exposure and wound failure, while those treated with the macroporous membrane remained submerged during the entire healing period. Therefore, it can be concluded that the use of a macroporous membrane may support flap survival during the healing period by enhancing vascularization.[19,20,22]

Enhancement of periodontal wound healing/regeneration has additionally been investigated by evaluating the use of agents that modify the root surface. In vitro studies used acidic or chelating agents for root surface demineralization or for the removal of bacterial endotoxins or the smear layer after root instrumentation, leading to exposure of the dentin tubules and the collagen matrix[23–26] and an enhanced adsorption/adhesion of the fibrin clot to the root surface.[27–29] Surface demineralization showed enhanced formation of new attachment compared with control sites in experimental animal studies,[9,30,31] but this effect has not been observed in clinical studies.[32–34] Moreover, wound healing in the form of a new connective tissue attachment and regeneration of all periodontal tissue (ie, alveolar bone, cementum, functionally oriented PDL) has been shown to be possible without removal of the smear layer or the exposure of the dentin collagen matrix and its growth factors.[17–20,22]

Taken together, observations from experimental studies point out the pivotal role of primary intention healing and space provision with barrier membranes without the need of tissue occlusion (ie, use of macroporous membranes) for achieving periodontal regeneration. Secondly, despite the positive effect of root surface biomodifying agents on fibrin clot adhesion/adsorption, their clinical use remains questionable.

BIOLOGIC CONCEPTS IN GTR

The concept of GTR was developed based on the early hypothesis by Melcher in 1976 and early animal experiments of Ellegaard et al[35,36] and Nielsen et al[37] suggesting that periodontal regeneration is induced by the cells originating from the PDL and not from the alveolar bone as previously believed.[13] As previously mentioned, this hypothesis was then confirmed in experimental studies by Karring et al.[14] Finally, in the early 1990s, it was definitively proven that the progenitor cells for regeneration of PDL derive from the PDL alone: in experimental studies in monkeys, formation of new PDL with inserting collagen fibers into new cementum and bone was observed after 12 months of healing when dental implants were inserted in alveolar bone in contact with root tips. Opposed to this, when implants were inserted just in bone, osseointegration (ie, implant surface in direct contact with bone) was obtained instead.[38–40]

Several further experimental studies investigated and confirmed the hypothesis that new attachment can be predictably achieved during healing by preventing the ingrowth of gingival connective tissue and epithelium to the root area, thus giving exclusivity to cells originating from the PDL.[18,41–48] In one of these studies in monkeys, cell-occlusive barrier membranes (cellulose acetate laboratory filter or ePTFE) were used to cover roots that had been previously infected (plaque accumulation for 6 months) and mechanically treated by scaling and root planing (SRP). In this study, significantly more new attachment was gained on the root surfaces covered with a membrane than the control sites that were not covered, which additionally showed signs of root resorption. However, bone was formed in both groups.[46]

A series of experimental studies on discriminating supra-alveolar defects in dogs were performed in 1991, demonstrating that undisturbed adhesion and maturation of a blood clot to the root surface is critical to attain periodontal regeneration. This ensures sufficient space for the periodontal tissue to regenerate and mature free of infection.[49] Thus, membranes have a rather protective role for the blood clot and wound maturation (ie, space provision, protection against tensile forces).

GTR was also shown to be successful in achieving predictable periodontal regeneration in experimental studies on clinical models for the treatment of intrabony[42,43,48,50] (Fig 2-3),

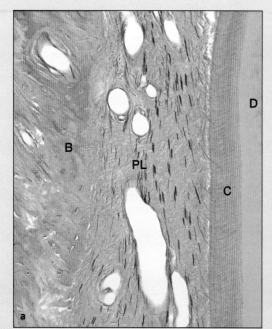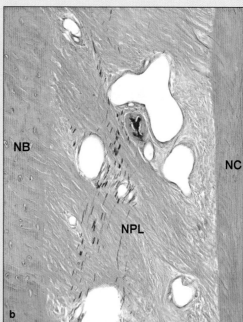

Fig 2-3 Light micrographs. *(a)* The genuine periodontal attachment with bone (B), periodontal ligament (PL), and cementum (C). *(b)* True periodontal regeneration with new attachment as demonstrated by new periodontal ligament (NPL) and fibers inserting into both new bone (NB) and new cementum (NC) after a regenerative GTR therapy with a bioresorbable membrane in a monkey tooth. D, dentin.

supra-alveolar,[18] recession,[44,45,51–59] and furcation-type defects.[41,47] Additionally, several reports provided human histologic evidence for the efficiency of GTR in regenerating lost periodontium (new cementum, new PDL, varying amounts of new alveolar bone) at sites affected by periodontitis and treated with SRP[17,60–63] (Fig 2-4).

The use of membranes in GTR

GTR was initially performed using nonresorbable membranes. Early reports evaluating the potential of various kinds of barrier membranes (eg, rubber dam, resin-ionomer) to regenerate periodontal tissues in intrabony defects showed only limited success.[64–66] It was therefore concluded that a membrane should be biocompatible, ensure tissue integration and space provisions, and be easy to clinically apply for periodontal regeneration to be predictably achieved.[67,68]

GTR was first shown to be successful in regenerating lost periodontal tissues in humans in a histologic study where teflon membranes (cellulose acetate laboratory filter called Millipore) were used to cover periodontally affected teeth after open flap debridement (OFD). The membranes were fixed to prevent any contact between the epithelium and

Fig 2-4 Micrographs at low *(a)* and high *(b)* magnifications illustrating periodontal regeneration on a human tooth after GTR therapy as demonstrated by the presence of new bone (NB), new periodontal ligament (NPL), and new cementum (NC) with inserting collagen fibers. A, artifact; D, dentin.

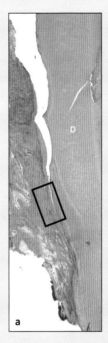 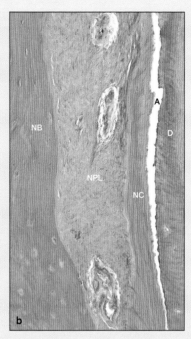

the gingival connective tissue and the root surfaces.[17] Later on, ePTFE (teflon) membranes were successfully used to regenerate lost periodontal tissues in various types of periodontal defects in both animal[11,42–43,45,46,69] and human studies.[50,56,61,70–72]

Despite successful regeneration with nonresorbable membranes, using them requires removal 4 to 6 weeks after implantation, which in turn may compromise the new regenerated tissue. A second surgical intervention is associated with bone resorption,[73] and wound healing by primary intention may not always be accomplished because it is not always possible to fully cover the newly formed periodontal tissues. In such cases, a 1.8- to 2.1-mm loss of clinical attachment level (CAL) was observed within 1 year after the second surgery.[74,75]

Considering these limitations of nonresorbable membranes, the use of synthetic (eg, oxidized cellulose mesh, calcium sulfate, polyurethanes)[76–79] or natural barrier resorbable membranes (human cadaveric dura mater, Cargile bovine membranes, laminar bone strips, type I and III porcine collagen)[80–83] have been implemented in GTR with various degrees of periodontal regeneration. Most investigated were membranes derived from collagen type I, PLA, and polyglycolic acid (PGA). The resorption process of collagen membranes relies on the enzymatic activity of the polymorphonuclear leucocytes and macrophages that infiltrate the wound during wound healing.[68,84] Additionally, PLA and

PGA membranes hydrolyze, and their degradation products are metabolized in the citric cycle.[85] However, timing is critical for these membranes to retain their physicochemical characteristics and their barrier function. For collagen membranes, this depends on the degree of collagen crosslinking; for PGA and PLA membranes, it depends on the relative concentration of the acids. Generally, a barrier function of at least 2 months should be assured.[86] Nonetheless, inferior outcomes for CAL gain and bone fill were obtained with these membranes in wide defects, where a longer period is likely required for regeneration than is needed with narrow defects.[87]

Several experimental[88–93] and human histologic studies[62,63,94] have predictably attained periodontal regeneration in various types of periodontal defects. These results have been confirmed clinically in further studies. In a systematic review and meta-analysis comparing the clinical efficiency after 6 months of GTR as opposed to OFD alone, a statistically significant added benefit for the use of ePTFE, polymeric, and collagen membranes was observed for CAL gain (1.61 mm, 0.92 mm, 0.95 mm) and PD reduction (1.41 mm, 0.89 mm, 1.06 mm), with no statistically significant differences among membranes.[95] Several studies report the long-term stability of clinical results after GTR with various types of resorbable membranes: PLA/citric acid ester copolymer,[96] polyglactin-910,[97] PLA/PGA,[98] and nonresorbable membranes.[57,99–101]

The role of grafting materials in periodontal regeneration

Bone grafts were introduced in periodontal regenerative therapy with the scope to enhance the regeneration of new bone, new PDL, and new root cementum either by osteoneogenesis (by releasing bone-forming cells), by osteoconduction (playing a role as a scaffold for bone formation), or by osteoinduction (by releasing bone-inducing substances). Grafts investigated for this purpose are divided according to their origin into autogenous grafts (derived from the same individual), allogeneic grafts (allografts, same species but different individuals), xenogeneic grafts (xenografts, from another species), and alloplastic materials (synthetic or anorganic material).

Autogenous grafts

Autogenous grafts are intended to maintain living cells that induce osteogenesis or osteoconduction. They can be divided in intra- and extraoral grafts depending on their origin. Despite the histologically proven regeneration of PDL, cementum, and alveolar bone in animal and human studies,[102–105] these grafts are not used in periodontal regenerative therapy because of the high rate of root resorption and ankylosis.[102–103]

Intraoral autogenous grafts are harvested from the retromolar mandibular region, edentulous space, chin area, and maxillary tuberosities. These grafts are gradually resorbed and replaced by new bone. Nonetheless, in a recent systematic review on human histologic studies, some of the included studies reported an encapsulation in bone or connective tissue and not complete resorption.[106] Controversial results for periodontal regeneration have been reported in human histologic studies: some reported complete to partial regeneration of the PDL, cementum, and alveolar bone,[107–110] while others noted a healing by means of long junctional epithelium.[111–113] Variable degrees of periodontal regeneration were also reported in a recent systematic review[106] where only 5 of the 10 included studies reported complete periodontal regeneration.[103,108,109,112,114] The others reported either partial regeneration and long junctional epithelium[110,111,113] or only long junctional epithelium.[115,116] Sculean et al[106] reported a residual defect depth of 3 mm and a new cementum and bone formation length of 1.9 mm (results from two studies).

Allografts

Allografts are an alternative to autogenous grafts. These do not require harvesting from a second surgical site and the associated risk of patient morbidity. Allografts derive from the same species (ie, humans) but are from a different individual (genetically different origin). Despite the rigorous processing of allografts, these still bear the risk of disease transmission and antigenicity. Two types of allograft have been investigated for the use in periodontal regenerative therapy: mineralized freeze-dried bone allograft (FDBA) and decalcified or demineralized freeze-dried bone allograft (DFDBA).

Although FDBA is supposed to promote regeneration through osteoconduction,[117] it was histologically shown to induce healing via long junctional epithelium with no periodontal regeneration.[118] Moreover, in a randomized controlled clinical trial, the use of FDBA in intrabony defects brought no additional improvement in terms of CAL gain or defect fill compared with OFD alone.[119]

DFDBA was shown to be osteogenic due to its bone morphogenetic proteins (BMPs), which are capable of inducing new bone formation.[120,121] Despite the fact that experimental studies showed no signs of periodontal regeneration,[122,123] DFDBA led to regeneration of all periodontal tissues in a human histologic study.[124,125] Moreover, two of the seven included studies in a recent systematic review[87] reported almost compete periodontal regeneration,[126,127] while six reported partial periodontal regeneration combined with formation of long junctional epithelium,[110,113,124–126,128] and only one study reported healing by long junctional epithelium alone.[129] These results corroborate those from several clinical studies that support the effective use of DFDBA in intrabony defects, reporting superior outcomes for CAL gain and defect fill compared with OFD alone.[130,131] Moreover, in a study evaluating the efficacy of autolysed antigen-extracted allogeneic bone for a longer observation period (ie, over 3 years), the statistically significantly higher amount of bone and CAL gain obtained 6 months postoperatively could be maintained up to 3 years (2.0 ± 0.7 mm vs 0.8 ± 0.5 mm).[130]

Xenografts

Bovine-derived xenografts (BDXs) were evaluated for periodontal regeneration in several animal and human histologic studies (Figs 2-5 to 2-7). Human histologic studies using BDX with and without a bioresorbable collagen membrane in intrabony defects resulted in the formation of new cellular cementum with functionally oriented inserting collagen fibers (PDL) on periodontally compromised root surfaces after 6 and 8 months.[80,132] Moreover, BDX particles were surrounded by newly formed bonelike tissue. In another study, BDX combined with collagen was shown to be efficient in treating human intrabony defects; after 9 months of healing, the biopsies provided evidence for formation of new cementum, new PDL, and new alveolar bone.[133] Comparable clinical results were reported by other authors for BDX and DFDBA in the treatment of intrabony defects[134] (see Figs 2-6 and 2-7).

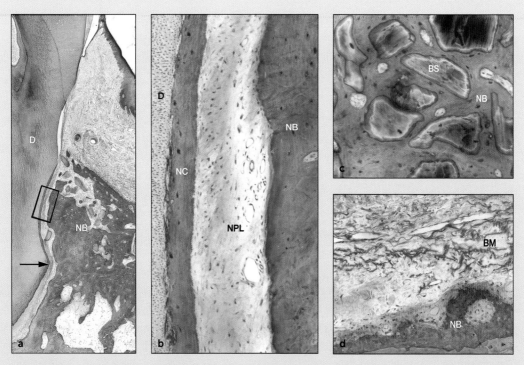

Fig 2-5 Light micrographs demonstrating periodontal regeneration in a dog tooth using the principle of GTR with a particulate xenogeneic bone substitute and a collagen barrier membrane. *(a)* Overview of the defect on the root surface. *(b)* Detail showing periodontal regeneration with new cementum (NC), new periodontal ligament (NPL), and new bone (NB). *(c)* Complete incorporation of the bone substitute (BS) particles in newly formed bone. *(d)* Residual collagen barrier membrane (BM) is present next to the surface of new bone. D, dentin.

Xenografts of coralline origin have also been investigated for periodontal regeneration. The natural coral can either be transformed into nonresorbable porous hydroxyapatite (HA) or into resorbable calcium carbonate. Controlled clinical trials showed better clinical outcomes (eg, probing depth [PD] reduction, CAL gain, defect fill) after grafting intrabony defects with coralline derivates compared with control sites,[135,136] and clinical outcomes were comparable with FDBA and DFDBA.[137,138] However, animal and human histologic studies revealed healing with a long junctional epithelium, encapsulation of the graft particles in connective tissue, and no periodontal regeneration.[139–141] These results are in line with those reported in the systematic review by Sculean et al.[106] Three of five studies reporting human histologic and histomorphometric results showed periodontal regeneration.[142–144] In an additional study, healing was described as a combination of periodontal regeneration and long junctional epithelium.[130] The only study that treated intrabony defects with coralline HA did not report any information related to the type of healing.[134] New bone was observed in direct contact with the graft particles in all studies. However, in some cases, the graft particles were observed encapsulated in connective tissue.

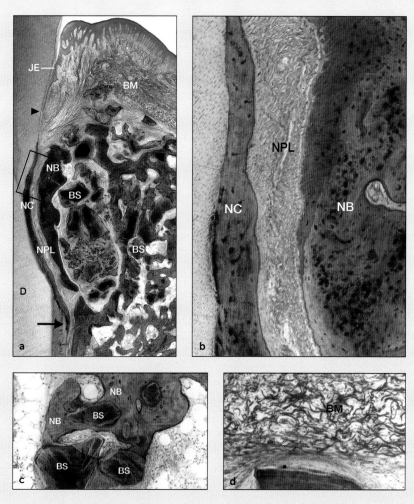

Fig 2-6 Light micrographs demonstrating periodontal regeneration in a human tooth using the principle of GTR with a particulate xenogeneic bone substitute combined with autogenous bone and a collagen barrier membrane. *(a)* Overview of the defect on the root surface. *(b)* Detail showing periodontal regeneration with new cementum (NC), new periodontal ligament (NPL), and new bone (NB). *(c)* Complete incorporation of the bone substitute (BS) particles in newly formed bone. *(d)* Residual collagen barrier membrane (BM) is present next to the surface of the bone substitute. D, dentin; JE, junctional epithelium.

Fig 2-7 Light micrograph illustrating the integration of xenogeneic bone substitute (BS) particles in newly formed bone (NB) after a GTR therapy with a collagen barrier membrane in a periodontal defect on a human tooth.

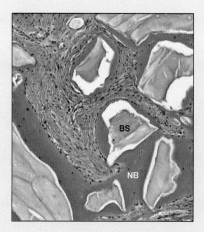

Alloplastic materials

Alloplastic grafts (eg, HA, β-tricalcium phosphate [β-TCP], polymers, bioactive glasses) are synthetically created, inorganic, biocompatible, and/or bioactive, and these types of grafts play an osteoconductive role in regeneration.[145–147]

Hydroxyapatite. HA may be used in either resorbable or nonresorbable form and has been shown to result in formation of a long junctional epithelium, encapsulation of the graft particles in connective tissue, and minimal bone formation in the vicinity of the bony walls.[143,148–150] Despite the lack of periodontal regeneration, results from clinical studies report better results regarding PD reductions, CAL gain, and defect fill than nongrafted defects.[151–154] Results were even comparable with autogenous bone spongiosa[155] or BDX.[156] On the other hand, systematic reviews showed controversial results for the use of alloplastic grafts.[157]

β-TCP. β-TCP is another synthetic alloplastic graft evaluated for periodontal regeneration. Despite the fact that several clinical studies reported significant CAL gain and defect fill after grafting of intrabony defects with β-TCP,[158–160] animal and human histologic reports described either quick resorption of β-TCP or an encapsulation of the graft particles in connective tissue, with seldom and minimal formation of new cementum and new bone.[148,161,162]

Polymers. Polymers are used in periodontal regenerative therapy as nonresorbable calcium hydroxide-coated copolymer of the polymethyl methacrylate (PMMA), polyhydroxyethyl methacrylate (PHEMA, also referred to as hard tissue replacement [HTR] polymer), or as resorbable polylactic acid. Neither histologic nor clinical results support its use in periodontal regeneration: healing resulted in encapsulation of HTR particles in connective tissue,[129,163,164] and clinically, no improvements for PD reduction or CAL gain were observed in grafted sites compared with nongrafted sites.[165–167]

Bioactive glasses. Bioactive glasses contain silicone dioxide (SiO_2), sodium oxide (Na_2O) and phosphorus pentoxide (P_2O_5) and can be realized in a resorbable and nonresorbable form. Despite the fact that animal studies have provided evidence for their good osteoconductive properties and their support in regenerating lost root cementum, PDL, and alveolar bone,[168] human histologic studies showed less promising results (Fig 2-8). Good clinical results regarding PD reductions and CAL gain were observed, but the healing was characterized by long junctional epithelium and encapsulation of the graft particles in connective tissue.[169,170] Moreover, clinical studies failed to consistently show better results in grafted sites with bioactive glasses compared with OFD alone.[171,172]

In a recent systematic review on human histologic studies, 10 studies that used alloplastic graft materials for the treatment of intrabony defects were included.[106] Histologic/histomorphometric analysis evidenced healing with formation of minimal bone and long junctional epithelium with encapsulation of the grafts. Even studies reporting on longer healing periods (eg, 18 to 30 months) described the presence of nonresorbed graft particles and their encapsulation in a fibrous tissue.[71,129,164]

Fig 2-8 Micrographs at low *(a)* and high *(b)* magnifications of human tooth root after therapy with Emdogain (Botiss) plus PerioGlas (NovaBone). There is only minimal periodontal regeneration, and the synthetic bone substitute particles are not integrated in new bone (NB). Instead, they are encapsulated by fibrous tissue (FT). The *arrow* indicates the bottom of the defect. A, artifact; D, dentin; G, gingiva; NC, new cementum; OB, old bone; PG, PerioGlas.

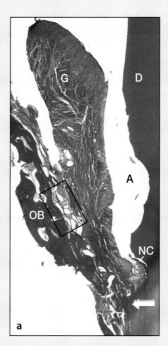
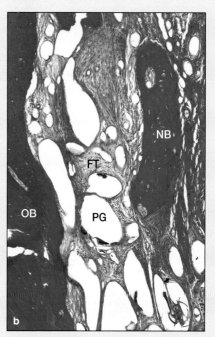

PERIODONTAL REGENERATION WITH BIOACTIVE AGENTS AND GROWTH FACTORS

Enamel matrix derivative

Proteins secreted during tooth development by the Hertwig epithelial root sheath layer are called *enamel matrix proteins* (EMPs). These play a major role in the development of acellular root cementum,[173,174] the most important tissue for tooth attachment to the alveolar bone.[175] EMPs consist of 90% amelogenins and 10% tuftelin, proline-rich nonamelogenins, and other serum proteins.[176] Amelogenins are very old EMPs (ie, over 100 million years),[177] hydrophobic, and insoluble at physiologic pH and body temperature; they self-assemble into aggregates of various sizes depending on the surrounding temperature.[176,178,179] They represent 90% of the enamel matrix and have been conserved well over time, showing just very small differences between amelogenins of various species (for example, porcine amelogenins are repeatedly used in humans).[176,180] Several experimental studies in rats, pigs, and monkeys provided evidence that an increase in amelogenin during tooth development plays an important role in the formation of acellular cementum.[175]

Based on these observations, it was assumed that amelogenins may promote regeneration of lost periodontal tissues by mimicking their development, and later experimental and clinical studies provided evidence that EMPs support periodontal regeneration.[75,181–185] For clinical implementation, enamel matrix derivative (EMD) was extracted and purified from the porcine enamel matrix of the premolar and molar crowns from 6-month-old pigs and combined with a vehicle of propylene glycol alginate (PPGA); thus Emdogain (previously Biora AB, then Straumann, now Botiss) was developed.[181] PPGA was chosen as a vehicle because amelogenins become soluble in an acidic or alkaline medium and low temperature and therefore dissolve in the PPGA solution (6% PPGA, acid pH of 3.2). In physiologic conditions (pH 7.4, temperature 35°C), the viscosity of Emdogain decreases, the PPGA vehicle is rinsed away within hours, and the amelogenins (ie, EMDs) have been shown to remain on the root surfaces up to 4 weeks.[181,186] Therefore, when applied surgically, amelogenin aggregates from the root surface come in close vicinity with connective tissue cells of the repositioned flap, representing a basic step in periodontal regeneration.[187]

Effects of EMD on periodontal tissues and evidence for periodontal regeneration

In vitro studies

The mechanisms of EMD on periodontal tissues including PDL, gingival fibroblasts, and bone cells were investigated in multiple in vitro experiments. Results from in vitro studies showed that EMD sustains fibroblast proliferation, inhibits epithelial cell proliferation, and increases protein synthesis and formation of mineralized nodules in PDL fibroblasts.[181,182] By inhibiting epithelial cell proliferation and the release of autocrine growth factors from PDL fibroblasts, EMD promotes proliferation of mesenchymal stem cells (MSCs).[188,189] Other experimental studies showed that EMD stimulated proliferation of PDL fibroblasts; had no effects on the adhesions, migration, and expression of type I collagen[190]; and may contain mitogenic factors, transforming growth factor β (TGF-β), and growth factors of the BMP family, therefore exerting a positive effect on fibroblast proliferation and mineralization during periodontal regeneration.[191–193] Despite the fact that metalloendoprotease and serine activities as well as growth factor activity were evidenced in EMD,[191–194] neither growth factors nor attachment proteins or other matrix proteins were detectable.[182,194] Further studies showed that EMD increased the osteogenic potential of bone marrow and formation of mineralized nodules[195] and has an impact on the differentiation of MSCs into osteoblasts and chondroblasts.[182,188,196,197]

In studies on human fibroblasts, EMD stimulated the alkaline phosphatase activity, fibroblast proliferation, and differentiation to cementoblasts.[198] EMDs were shown to positively influence fibroblast viability, proliferation, and attachment to previously diseased root surfaces[199]; additionally, they sustain the messenger RNA (mRNA) synthesis of some matrix proteins and hyaluronan synthesis in the gingival and periodontal fibroblasts, with a stronger effect on those of PDL origin.[196–200] On epithelial cells, it was shown that EMD exercises a cytotoxic effect[201] and an osteopromotive (and not osteoinductive) effect at a certain dosage.[202]

Further in vitro studies provided evidence that EMD has a positive effect on wound healing by exerting inhibitory effects on various genes involved in early inflammatory phases in wound healing and stimulating those involved in repair and growth.[203] Moreover, other studies showed that EMD accelerates wound closure in rabbits[204] and has angiogenetic effects positively influencing wound healing.[205] Additionally, EMD and PPGA carriers have strong antibacterial effects,[206] inhibiting the growth of *Aggregatibacter actinomycetem-comitans*, *Porphyromonas gingivalis*, and *Prevotella intermedia*[207,208] without influencing gram-positive bacteria.[209] On the other hand, *P gingivalis* also suppresses the effect of EMD on PDL cells.[210] EMD seems to also systemically inhibit the release of tumor necrosis factor α (TNF-α) and interleukin 8 (IL-8), pointing to potential anti-inflammatory properties.

Histologic animal and human studies

In 1997, the first animal and human histologic studies provided evidence for periodontal regeneration after application of Emdogain.[183,211] Hammarström et al[211] showed formation of new root cementum (acellular cementum), new PDL, and new alveolar bone in a buccal dehiscence model in monkeys treated with EMD, while control sites (coronally repositioned flap) healed with formation of long junctional epithelium. Additionally, sites treated with EMD showed no signs of root resorption, as opposed to control sites.[211]

In the same year, the first human histologic evidence for periodontal regeneration with EMD was also provided, showing that the application of EMD on a previously debrided and etched root surface in an experimental defect led to formation of new acellular cementum with functionally oriented inserting collagen fibers and new alveolar bone.[183] Another human histologic study also reported promising results for the treatment of intrabony defects with EMD. Three of the ten defects analyzed showed full periodontal regeneration, three demonstrated healing with new cementum and inserting collagen fibers, and the remaining four healed with a long junctional epithelium.[212]

These observations were followed and supported by further histologic studies: Sculean et al[213] found formation of oxytalan fibers (PDL fibers) within the newly formed PDL after application of EMD or GTR in single-wall intrabony and furcation grade III defects in monkeys; these were functionally oriented (apico-occlusal direction) and present only in association with newly formed cementum.[213] In this study, EMD was shown to provide a similar amount of new attachment compared with GTR (Fig 2-9). In a subsequent human histologic study on 14 patients, similar amounts of new attachment (ie, new collagen fibers inserting in new cementum) were detected histomorphometrically after application of EMD or GTR in advanced intrabony defects (PD ≥ 11 mm); nonetheless, significantly less new bone was obtained in sites treated with EMD alone (0.9 ± 1.0 mm) than with GTR (2.1 ± 1.0 mm)[63] (Fig 2-10). These results were in line with another human multicenter study, where similar significant amounts of new attachment (ie, new cementum with inserting collagen fibers) were observed both with EMD and with GTR. Nonetheless, statistically significant new bone was observed only in the defects treated with GTR.[214]

In another human histologic study (two patients with chronic periodontitis and deep intrabony defects), Emdogain was shown to induce formation of new cementum with inserting collagen fibers after a healing period of 6 months. In one defect, regeneration of alveolar bone was also observed.[215] Results from human immunohistologic studies provided evidence that EMD remains on the root surfaces for up to 4 weeks.[186,216] Moreover, the new tissues that formed 2 to 6 weeks after EMD application in intrabony defects were characterized by a thick, collagenous, electron-dense organic material. Numerous large cells were

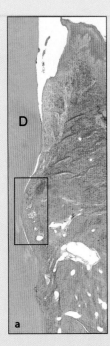
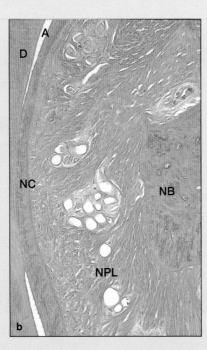

Fig 2-9 Micrographs illustrating periodontal regeneration on a monkey tooth at low *(a)* and high *(b)* magnifications after regenerative therapy with Emdogain. New bone (NB), new periodontal ligament (NPL), and new cementum (NC) with inserting collagen fibers demonstrate new attachment to the treated root surface. A, artifact; D, dentin.

embedded in a partially mineralized collagenous matrix.[217,218] Thus, after treatment with EMD on previously scaled root surfaces, new mineralized connective tissue may be formed as well as a bonelike tissue similar to the cellular intrinsic fiber cementum. No periodontal regeneration was observed when EMD was applied nonsurgically.[219,220]

Further research was undertaken on whether the combination of GTR and EMD would provide any additional improvement in regenerating lost periodontal tissues as opposed to EMD or GTR alone. Acute fenestration-type defects were surgically created in monkeys. Healing after application of EMD or GTR consistently resulted in new connective tissue attachment and new bone formation in defects treated with GTR, as opposed to those treated with EMD or a coronally advanced flap alone, where periodontal regeneration was observed to a varying extent.[221] After this, the combination of EMD and GTR was evaluated in two subsequent histologic studies in monkeys in recession-type and intrabony defects (surgically created and exposed to plaque accumulation).[48,221] After 5 months of healing, the defects treated with EMD alone showed periodontal regeneration to a varying extent, while it was noticed consistently in defects treated with GTR without membrane exposure. Nonetheless, the combination of GTR and EMD provided no additional effect.[48]

In mandibular grade III furcation defects in monkeys, GTR and EMD alone or combined were compared with OFD.[222] Healing resulted in periodontal regeneration (ie, new cementum with inserting collagen fibers and new bone) in defects treated with GTR and EMD combined with GTR where the membrane was unexposed. Periodontal regeneration was

Fig 2-10 Light micrographs at low *(a)* and high *(b)* magnifications demonstrating periodontal regeneration on human tooth roots after periodontal regenerative therapy with Emdogain. New bone (NB), new periodontal ligament (NPL), and new cementum (NC) with inserting collagen fibers are present. D, dentin; OC, old cementum.

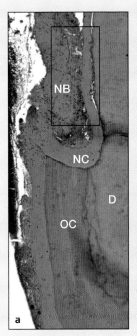
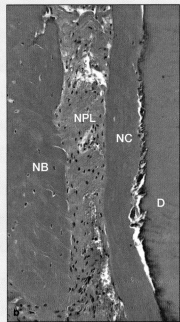

observed to a varying extent at sites treated with EMD alone and only limited at control sites (ie, only new attachment and bone formation).[222] In another histomorphometric study evaluating the effect of EMD with and without GTR in grade II furcation defects in dogs, EMD resulted in significant amounts of periodontal regeneration with a negative effect when combined with GTR. Control sites treated with OFD alone healed with long junctional epithelium and limited bone formation.[223]

Controversial results have been reported for periodontal regeneration when EMD was combined with xenografts. In a human histologic study in three patients, intrabony defects were treated with a BDX (one defect) or with EMD combined with BDX (two defects).[132] The histologic analyses after 6 months of healing showed formation of new attachment (ie, new cementum with functionally oriented collagen fibers) and new bone in all teeth. BDX particles were surrounded by bonelike tissue with no contact between the BDX particles or with the root surfaces.[132]

In a histologic study in 16 patients with advanced intrabony defects where EMD was nonsurgically applied after SRP, healing in the test group resulted in long junctional epithelium without signs of periodontal regeneration similar to the control group (SRP alone).[219] EMD can be detectable up to 4 weeks on previously diseased and scaled root surfaces.

Taken together, results from animal and human histologic studies indicate that the surgical application of EMD in periodontal regenerative surgery promotes formation of new cementum, new alveolar bone, and new PDL fibers in recession-type and intrabony defects.

Growth factors

Growth and differentiation factors have been investigated for their potential support in periodontal wound healing and regeneration. The mechanism is based on their involvement in the regulation of chemotaxis, proliferation, differentiation, and synthesis of the cell matrix.[224] They bind to specific cell-surface receptors, transmit signals to the cell nucleus by means of intracellular signal transduction pathways, and activate specific target genes to regulate the cell activity and phenotype.[225–227] Growth factors may locally or systemically affect the target cells in various ways: autocrine, paracrine, intracrine, juxtacrine, or endocrine.[227] Growth factors themselves are regulated by complex interactions with other growth factors, enzymes, proteins, and regulatory factors.[228,229] For clinical use, growth factors have been used with various delivery systems: tissue derivatives (eg, bone, dermal collagen, inorganic bone), synthetic products (eg, ceramic and polymeric matrices), genes, and living cells.

This section presents only the growth factors that have been most investigated for periodontal regeneration.

Platelet-derived growth factor (PDGF)

PDGF is secreted by platelet α-granules and by various cells such as macrophages, fibroblasts, myocytes, endothelial, glial, and bone marrow hematopoietic cells.[230,231] It can be found in four isoforms—A, B, C, and D—and two homodimers of PDGF-A (AA) and -B (BB).[232,233]

PDGF-A, -B, and -AB have been investigated for their effect on periodontal regeneration. Promising in vitro results bring evidence that these isoforms support and promote chemotaxis, proliferation, and the protein synthesis of the gingival and PDL fibroblasts.[234,235] They have an anabolic effect on osteocytes[236,237] and downregulate alkaline phosphatase, osteocalcin, and osteopontin.[238,239] PDGF-B stimulates both human PDL cell proliferation[240] and cementoblast mitogenesis.[241]

Preclinical animal studies evaluated its application in acute and chronic defects. In a study in dogs, PDGF applied in a carrier matrix alone or with GTR in periodontal fenestration–type defects showed enhanced proliferation of the fibroblasts in the early healing phase (1 to 7 days postsurgically).[242] In another study in dogs, PDGF-B and GTR showed significantly more bone fill, faster periodontal healing, and almost complete regeneration in all grade III furcation defects compared with GTR alone, which resulted in complete regeneration only at the defects located at the second premolar.[243] Moreover, in an experimental study in monkeys, significantly more bone fill and new attachment were observed in chronic periodontal defects treated with PDGF-B as opposed to the control group (vehicle alone).[244] Human histologic studies evaluating the use of recombinant human PDFG-BB (rhPDGF-BB) at various concentrations (0.5, 1.0, 5.0 mg/mL) in an allogeneic DFDBA matrix for deep intrabony and furcation defects reported a variable degree of new periodontal attachment in four of the six intrabony defects and in all four furcation defects.[245,246] Nonetheless, no control sites had been used, and therefore the real advantage of PDGF is questionable. When rhPDGF-BB was used with a β-TCP carrier, only limited regeneration was obtained (12 out of 16 defects) with new bone formation only adjacent to the bony walls.[247] Thus, the successful use of PDGF in periodontal regeneration is questionable.

Insulin-like growth factors (IGFs)

IGFs include several growth factors like insulin, relaxin, IGF-1, and IGF-2 and are involved in chemotaxis, proliferation, differentiation, transformation, antiapoptosis, and similar functions.[248] IGF-1 has been shown to enhance the proliferation and migration of PDL and gingival fibroblasts,[249] to stimulate bone formation and synthesis of type I collagen,[250] to upregulate the gene coding for bone-associated proteins,[251] to increase the cortical and trabecular bone formation, to stimulate osteoblast proliferation, and to decrease the osteo-clast activity in both rat and human in vitro studies.[252] However, no promising results were obtained in experimental histologic studies. In an experimental study in monkeys, only limited regeneration was observed after 12 months of healing following the application of IGF-1 in chronic periodontal defects with no detectable difference to the control group.[244] Similar results were reported in a dog study with only limited new bone formation.[253]

Nonetheless, promising results were obtained when IGF-1 was combined with PDGF. Significantly more new bone and cementum formation were observed after 2 to 5 weeks of healing in naturally occurring periodontal defects in a dog study when rhPDGF-B was combined with IGF-1 when compared with the control sites.[254,255] Similar findings were seen in an experimental study in monkeys, where the combination group showed the most periodontal regeneration compared with the single use of the growth factors or the carrier group.[244] These studies were followed by a clinical study evaluating the combination of rhPDGF-BB and IGF-1 in various concentrations: only rhPDGF-BB/IGF-1 at 150/150 µg/mL showed significant bone fill compared with the controls and to the tested combination in a concentration of 50/50 mg/mL.[256] The effects of PDGF and IGF-1 on periodontal regeneration were not further investigated.

Fibroblast growth factors (FGFs)

FGFs are polypeptides and represent more than 20 forms with similar structural characteristics and various biologic effects on cells. One main FGF is the basic FGF (bFGF) or FGF-2. bFGF promotes angiogenesis, cell proliferation, and synthesis of noncollagenous proteins.[257] It can be found in the bone matrix influencing bone growth.[258] In the oral cavity, bFGF seems to be produced by endothelial cells and PDL fibroblasts.[259] In vitro studies pointed out that bFGF promotes the proliferation of PDL cells but inhibits their differentiation[260]; moreover, it stimulates the migration of PDL and gingival fibroblasts, chemotaxis, and several other biologic effects.[224,261] In preclinical animal studies, various concentrations of bFGF were applied in surgically created grade II furcation defects in dogs and monkeys. After a healing period of 6 weeks in dogs and 8 weeks in monkeys, there was a significantly greater periodontal regeneration with a twofold increase in cementum and bone for the high dose.[260] No ankylosis, root resorption, or epithelial downgrowth were observed. These results were supported by subsequent similar studies.[262,263] Moreover, bFGF seems to result in additional regeneration when combined with GTR as opposed to sites treated with GTR alone for the treatment of mandibular grade III furcation defects in dogs.[264] Other experimental animal studies suggested a positive effect on the resolution of anky-lotic signs[265]; however, these are just speculations based on observed healing patterns in animals. Despite these promising preclinical results, bFGF has not yet been implemented in a clinical protocol with predictable results.

Transforming growth factor β (TGF-β)

TGF-β is represented by a series of polypeptide growth factors involved in embryogenesis and afterward in the regulation of inflammation, immune response and wound healing.[266] There are five TGF-β isoforms (TGF-β1–5) with TGF-β1 being identical in several species. TGF-β is synthetized by many cells, like macrophages, fibroblasts, tumor cells, and platelets, and it may be found in platelets, cartilage bone, and dentin. Several in vitro studies provided evidence that TGF-β promotes the synthesis of the PDL extracellular matrix as well as the PDL mitogenesis and proliferation.[234,235,249,207] Additionally, TGF-β may play an important role in the development and maturation of the periodontium,[267] in periodontal wound healing,[268] and in inhibiting epithelial cell proliferation.[254] Further biologic effects on periodontal tissues include chemotaxis, synthesis of type I collagen, fibronectin, osteonectin, and bone matrix deposition.[269,270] TGF-β seems to stimulate osteoblasts on one hand and inhibit osteoclast formation and bone resorption on the other hand. It is richly formed during bone resorption and is supposed to play an important regulatory role in bone remodeling.[271] A helpful resource with more detailed information is the chapter by Stavropoulos and Wikesjö in *Periodontal Regenerative Therapy* (Quintessence, 2010).[224]

Based on the observed biologic effects of TGF-β in in vitro studies, further experimental studies on sheep and dog models have been performed to evaluate the effects of TGF-β in periodontal regeneration and wound healing. Promising results were obtained when TGF-β1 was used either with a carrier or combined with GTR in surgically created mandibular premolar grade II furcation defects in a sheep model. After 6 weeks of healing, significantly greater bone formation and new cementum were observed in the sites treated with TGF-β1 as opposed to the control sites (carrier alone). The combination of GTR and TGF-β1 showed more bone formation than TGF-β1 alone.[272] Contrary to these results, in another study in a dog model, only limited to no formation of new cementum and minimal bone formation in the apical aspect of the defects was observed when rhTGF-β1 (20 mg/defects) was applied with a carrier of $CaCO_3$/hydroxyethyl or combined with GTR as opposed to carrier alone, or carrier and/or GTR, or GTR alone.[273–275] It seemed that rhTGF-β1 accelerated the resorption of the carrier, proving its biologic activity.[276] Nonetheless, it is debatable that the carrier may negatively affect the possible biologic effects of TGF-β1 on periodontal wound healing and regeneration. Therefore, TGF-β1 cannot yet be recommended for periodontal regeneration.

Bone morphogenetic proteins (BMPs)

BMPs belong to a TGF-β superfamily and have been shown to play a key role in bone induction.[277] The BMP family includes more than 20 types of proteins with homodimeric or heterodimeric structure and are found in multiple species (eg, fruit flies, frogs, mammals). BMPs are involved in skeletal modeling, tissue morphogenesis, organogenesis, chemotaxis regulation, mitosis, cartilage differentiation, differentiation of MSCs into various cell types, and similar functions.[278,279] For more detailed information about the structure and function of BMPs, see the chapter on growth factors by Drs Stavropoulos and Wikesjö in Dr Sculean's *Periodontal Regenerative Therapy*.[224]

Some BMPs have been investigated for periodontal wound healing/regeneration: BMP-2, -3 (osteogenin), -4, -6, -7 (osteogenic protein 1: OP-1), -12 (growth differentiation factor 7: GDF-7), -14 (GDF-5 or cartilage-derived morphogenetic protein 1: CDMP-1).[224] Based on findings from various in vitro experiments and studies in mice, it is suggested that BMPs are involved in all stages of tooth morphogenesis: BMP-2, -4, -5, -7, -13, and -14 regulate dentin and enamel formation, while BMP-3, -7, -12, -13, and -14 are involved in cementogenesis and PDL formation. BMP-2 may also play an important role in alveolar bone formation.[280–282]

BMP-2

* *rhBMP-2 (0.2 mg/mL) carried on bioresorbable poly (lactic-co-glycolic acid) (PLGA) microparticles and autogenous blood:* Led to significantly greater alveolar bone and cementum formation compared with carriers alone in supra-alveolar periodontal defects in dogs (healing period of 8 weeks).[283,284]
* *rhBMP-2 (0.2 mg/mL) carried on allogeneic canine demineralized bone matrix (DBM/ type I absorbable collagen sponge (ACS)/bioresorbable PLGA microparticles/PLA granules:* Resulted in substantial bone regeneration with varying bone volume and density, cementum formation, and ankylosis according to the used carrier in the critical-size supra-alveolar periodontal defect model in dogs.[285]
* *rhBMP-2 carried on ACS with or without perforated ePTFE membrane:* Showed a significantly greater amount of bone formation when combined with a membrane as opposed to rhBMP-2 alone or carrier alone in supra-alveolar periodontal defects in dogs. Cementum formation was similar at sites treated with rhBMP-2, and functionally oriented PDL fibers were seen inconsistently.[22,286]
* *rhBMP-2:* Resulted in greater amounts of new bone and cementum compared with control sites in surgically created or chronic defects in dogs,[22,283,285,286] monkeys,[287] cats,[265] and rats.[288]

BMP-3 (osteogenin)

* *BMP-3 combined with DFDBA/bovine tendon-derived collagen matrix*: Led to significantly higher amounts of periodontal regeneration in submerged intrabony periodontal defects in humans compared with carrier alone (tendon-derived collagen).[127]
* *BMP-3 (with small amounts of BMP-2 and BMP-7) combined with a collagenous matrix carrier:* Resulted in significantly greater amounts of periodontal regeneration (Sharpey fibers inserting in new cementum) and new bone formation compared with carrier alone in surgically created mandibular molar grade II furcation defects in monkeys.[289]

BMP-6

* Limited experimental observations in rats provide evidence for periodontal regeneration in periodontal fenestration defects.[290]

BMP-7 (OP-1)

* *OP-1 (concentrations of 0, 100, and 500 μg/g) carried on bovine bone insoluble collagen matrix:* Resulted in significant amounts of new cementum with inserting Sharpey fibers as opposed to controls in surgically created mandibular grade II furcation defects in monkeys.[291]

- *rhOP-1 (concentrations of 0.5 and 2.5 mg/g) carried on collagen matrix:* Showed significantly greater amounts of periodontal regeneration (functionally oriented Sharpey fibers inserting in new bone and new cementum) in grade II furcations in monkeys.[292]
- *rhOP-1:* Showed greater periodontal regeneration compared with sham surgery or carrier control in large supra-alveolar defects in dogs. Signs of ankylosis and root resorption were also present.[293]
- *rhOP-1 combined with rhBMP-2 in 100 µg/g collagen matrix*: Showed no additional enhancement regarding formation of new bone or new attachment compared with rhOP-1 alone or rhBMP-2 alone. rhOP-1 alone resulted in significantly greater amounts of new cementum, while rhBMP-2 alone showed significantly greater amounts of new bone compared with the other groups.[294]

BMP-12 (GDF-7)

- *GDF-7:* Led to formation of functionally oriented PDL inserting in new bone and cementum in supra-alveolar periodontal defects in humans.[295]

BMP-14 (GDF-5)

- *rhBMP-14 concentration 20 µg carred on β-TCP or in 1, 20, or 100 µg carried on ACS:* Led to significantly greater periodontal regeneration (higher amounts of new bone and cementum, functionally oriented PDL) compared with carriers alone or sham surgery in surgically created mandibular single-wall intrabony periodontal defects in dogs. rhBMP-14/β-TCP provided significantly greater amounts of new bone than the combination with the collagen sponge carrier.[296]
- *rhGDF-5/βhGDF:* Led to significantly higher amounts of new bone and cementum compared with a commercially available rhPDGF/β (GEM 21S, Lynch Biologics) in single-wall intrabony periodontal defects in dogs.[297]
- *rhGDF-5/βhGDF:* Resulted in significantly higher amounts (ie, almost three times more) new alveolar bone compared with OFD alone on advanced intrabony human periodontal defects.[298,299]

Taken together, these studies provide promising results for the role of some growth factors in periodontal wound healing and regeneration. Nonetheless, the choice of an appropriate delivery system may negatively influence the outcomes, and no optimal carrier has yet been identified.

REFERENCES

1. Wikesjö UM, Polimeni G, Xiropaids AV, Stavropoulos A. Periodontal wound healing/regeneration. In: Sculean A (ed). Periodontal Regenerative Therapy, vol 1. London: Quintessence, 2010:25–45.
2. Clark RAF. Wound repair: Overview and general considerations. In: Clark RAF, Henson PM (eds). The Molecular and Cellular Biology of Wound Repair, ed 2. New York: Plenum, 1996:3–50.
3. Jennings RW, Hunt TK. Overview of postnatal wound healing. In: Adzick NS, Longaker MT (eds). Fetal Wound Healing. New York: Elsevier, 1992:25–52.
4. Wikesjö UM, Crigger M, Nilvéus R, Selvig KA. Early healing events at the dentin-connective tissue interface. Light and transmission electron microscopy observations. J Periodontol 1991;62:5–14.

5. Grzesik WJ, Narayanan AS. Cementum and periodontal wound healing and regeneration. Crit Rev Oral Biol Med 2002;13:474–484.
6. Stahl SS, Slavkin HC, Yamada L, Levine S. Speculations about gingival repair. J Periodontol 1972;43:395–402.
7. Wikesjö UM, Selvig KA. Periodontal wound healing and regeneration. Periodontol 2000 1999;19:21–39.
8. Hiatt WH, Stallard RE, Butler ED, Badgett B. Repair following mucoperiosteal flap surgery with full gingival retention. J Periodontol 1968;39:11–16.
9. Polson AM, Proye MP. Fibrin linkage: A precursor for new attachment. J Periodontol 1983;54:141–147.
10. Wikesjö UM, Claffey N, Egelberg J. Periodontal repair in dogs. Effect of heparin treatment of the root surface. J Clin Periodontol 1991;18:60–64.
11. Haney JM, Nilvéus RE, McMillan PJ, Wikesjö UM. Periodontal repair in dogs: Expanded polytetrafluoroethylene barrier membranes support wound stabilization and enhance bone regeneration. J Periodontol 1993;64:883–890.
12. Wikesjö UM, Nilvéus R. Periodontal repair in dogs: Effect of wound stabilization on healing. J Periodontol 1990;61:719–724.
13. Melcher AH. On the repair potential of periodontal tissues. J Periodontol 1976;47:256–260.
14. Karring T, Nyman S, Gottlow J, Laurell L. Development of the biological concept of guided tissue regeneration: Animal and human studies. Periodontol 2000 1993;1:26–35.
15. Karring T, Nyman S, Lindhe J. Healing following implantation of periodontitis affected roots into bone tissue. J Clin Periodontol 1980;7:96–105.
16. Nyman S, Karring T, Lindhe J, Plantén S. Healing following implantation of periodontitis-affected roots into gingival connective tissue. J Clin Periodontol 1980;7:394–401.
17. Nyman S, Lindhe J, Karring T, Rylander H. New attachment following surgical treatment of human periodontal disease. J Clin Periodontol 1982;9:290 296.
18. Sigurdsson TJ, Hardwick R, Bogle GC, Wikesjö UM. Periodontal repair in dogs: Space provision by reinforced ePTFE membranes enhances bone and cementum regeneration in large supra alveolar defects. J Periodontol 1994;65:350–356.
19. Wikesjö UM, Lim WH, Thomson RC, Hardwick WR. Periodontal repair in dogs: Gingival tissue occlusion, a critical requirement for GTR? J Clin Periodontol 2003;30:655–664.
20. Wikesjö UM, Lim WH, Thomson RC, Cook AD, Wozney JM, Hardwick WR. Periodontal repair in dogs: Evaluation of a bioabsorbable space-providing macro-porous membrane with recombinant human bone morphogenetic protein-2. J Periodontol 2003;74:635–647.
21. Karaki R, Kubota K, Hitaka M, Yamaji S, Kataoka R, Yamamoto H. Effect of gum-expanding-mesh on the osteogenesis of surgical bony defects [in Japanese]. Nihon Shishubyo Gakkai Kaishi 1984;26:516–522.
22. Wikesjö UM, Xiropaidis AV, Thomson RC, Cook AD, Selvig KA, Hardwick WR. Periodontal repair in dogs: rhBMP-2 significantly enhances bone formation under provisions for guided tissue regeneration. J Clin Periodontol 2003;30:705–714.
23. Blomlöf J, Lindskog S. Root surface texture and early cell and tissue colonization after different etching modalities. Eur J Oral Sci 1995;103:17–24.
24. Polson AM, Frederick GT, Ladenheim S, Hanes PJ. The production of a root surface smear layer by instrumentation and its removal by citric acid. J Periodontol 1984;55:443–446.
25. Wikesjö UM, Baker PJ, Christersson LA, et al. A biochemical approach to periodontal regeneration: Tetracycline treatment conditions dentin surfaces. J Periodontal Res 1986;21:322–329.
26. Trombelli L, Scabbia A, Zangari F, Griselli A, Wikesjö UM, Calura G. Effect of tetracycline HCl on periodontally-affected human root surfaces. J Periodontol 1995;66:685–691.
27. Baker DL, Seymour GJ. The possible pathogenesis of gingival recession. A histological study of induced recession in the rat. J Clin Periodontol 1976;3:208–219.
28. Baker DL, Stanley Pavlow SA, Wikesjö UM. Fibrin clot adhesion to dentin conditioned with protein constructs: An in vitro proof-of-principle study. J Clin Periodontol 2005;32:561–566.
29. Baker PJ, Rotch HA, Trombelli L, Wikesjö UM. An in vitro screening model to evaluate root conditioning protocols for periodontal regenerative procedures. J Periodontol 2000;71:1139–1143.
30. Nilvéus R, Egelberg J. The effect of topical citric acid application on the healing of experimental furcation defects in dogs. III. The relative importance of coagulum support, flap design and systemic antibiotics. J Periodontal Res 1980;15:551–560.
31. Wikesjö UM, Claffey N, Nilvéus R, Egelberg J. Periodontal repair in dogs: Effect of root surface treatment with stannous fluoride or citric acid on root resorption. J Periodontol 1991;62:180–184.
32. Mariotti A. Efficacy of chemical root surface modifiers in the treatment of periodontal disease. A systematic review. Ann Periodontol 2003;8:205–226.
33. Trombelli L, Scabbia A, Scapoli C, Calura G. Clinical effect of tetracycline demineralization and fibrin-fibronectin sealing system application on healing response following flap debridement surgery. J Periodontol 1996;67:688–693.
34. Trombelli L, Scabbia A, Wikesjö UM, Calura G. Fibrin glue application in conjunction with tetracycline root conditioning and coronally positioned flap procedure in the treatment of human gingival recession defects. J Clin Periodontol 1996;23:861–867.
35. Ellegaard B, Karring T, Löe H. The fate of vital and devitalized bone grafts in the healing of interradicular lesions. J Periodontal Res 1975;10:88–97.

36. Ellegaard B, Nielsen IM, Karring T. Composite jaw and iliac cancellous bone grafts in intrabony defects in monkeys. J Periodontal Res 1976;11:299–310.

37. Nielsen IM, Ellegaard B, Karring T. Kielbone in healing interradicular lesions in monkeys. J Periodontal Res 1980;15:328–337.

38. Buser D, Warrer K, Karring T. Formation of a periodontal ligament around titanium implants. J Periodontol 1990;61:597–601.

39. Buser D, Warrer K, Karring T, Stich H. Titanium implants with a true periodontal ligament: An alternative to osseointegrated implants? Int J Oral Maxillofac Implants 1990;5:113–116.

40. Warrer K, Karring T, Gotfredsen K. Periodontal ligament formation around different types of dental titanium implants. I. The self-tapping screw type implant system. J Periodontol 1993;64:29–34.

41. Caffesse RG, Dominguez LE, Nasjleti CE, Castelli WA, Morrison EC, Smith BA. Furcation defects in dogs treated by guided tissue regeneration (GTR). J Periodontol 1990;61:45–50.

42. Caffesse RG, Smith BA, Castelli WA, Nasjleti CE. New attachment achieved by guided tissue regeneration in beagle dogs. J Periodontol 1988;59:589–594.

43. Caton J, Wagener C, Polson A, et al. Guided tissue regeneration in interproximal defects in the monkey. Int J Periodontics Restorative Dent 1992;12:266–277.

44. Cortellini P, DeSanctis M, Pini Prato G, Baldi C, Clauser C. Guided tissue regeneration procedure using a fibrin-fibronectin system in surgically induced recession in dogs. Int J Periodontics Restorative Dent 1991;11:150–163.

45. Gottlow J, Karring T, Nyman S. Guided tissue regeneration following treatment of recession-type defects in the monkey. J Periodontol 1990;61:680–685.

46. Gottlow J, Nyman S, Karring T, Lindhe J. New attachment formation as the result of controlled tissue regeneration. J Clin Periodontol 1984;11:494–503.

47. Niederman R, Savitt ED, Heeley JD, Duckworth JE. Regeneration of furca bone using Gore-Tex periodontal material. Int J Periodontics Restorative Dent 1989;9:468–480.

48. Sculean A, Donos N, Brecx M, Reich E, Karring T. Treatment of intrabony defects with guided tissue regeneration and enamel-matrix-proteins. An experimental study in monkeys. J Clin Periodontol 2000;27:466–472.

49. Wikesjö UM, Nilvéus R. Periodontal repair in dogs. Healing patterns in large circumferential periodontal defects. J Clin Periodontol 1991;18:49–59.

50. Trombelli L, Kim CK, Zimmerman GJ, Wikesjö UM. Retrospective analysis of factors related to clinical outcome of guided tissue regeneration procedures in intrabony defects. J Clin Periodontol 1997;24:366–371.

51. Trombelli L, Schincaglia GP, Zangari F, Griselli A, Scabbia A, Calura G. Effects of tetracycline HCl conditioning and fibrin-fibronectin system application in the treatment of buccal gingival recession with guided tissue regeneration. J Periodontol 1995;66:313–320.

52. Trombelli L, Schincaglia GP, Scapoli C, Calura G. Healing response of human buccal gingival recessions treated with expanded polytetrafluoroethylene membranes. A retrospective report. J Periodontol 1995;66:14–22.

53. Trombelli L, Scabbia A, Tatakis DN, Checchi L, Calura G. Resorbable barrier and envelope flap surgery in the treatment of human gingival recession defects. Case reports. J Clin Periodontol 1998;25:24–29.

54. Trombelli L, Minenna L, Farina R, Scabbia A. Guided tissue regeneration in human gingival recessions. A 10-year follow-up study. J Clin Periodontol 2005;32:16–20.

55. Tatakis DN, Trombelli L. Gingival recession treatment: Guided tissue regeneration with bioabsorbable membrane versus connective tissue graft. J Periodontol 2000;71:299–307.

56. Trombelli L. Periodontal regeneration in gingival recession defects. Periodontol 2000 1999;19:138–150.

57. Scabbia A, Trombelli L. Long-term stability of the mucogingival complex following guided tissue regeneration in gingival recession defects. J Clin Periodontol 1998;25:1041–1046.

58. Trombelli L, Scabbia A, Tatakis DN, Calura G. Subpedicle connective tissue graft versus guided tissue regeneration with bioabsorbable membrane in the treatment of human gingival recession defects. J Periodontol 1998;69:1271–1277.

59. Trombelli L, Tatakis DN, Scabbia A, Zimmerman GJ. Comparison of mucogingival changes following treatment with coronally positioned flap and guided tissue regeneration procedures. Int J Periodontics Restorative Dent 1997;17:448–455.

60. Cortellini P, Clauser C, Prato GP. Histologic assessment of new attachment following the treatment of a human buccal recession by means of a guided tissue regeneration procedure. J Periodontol 1993;64:387–391.

61. Gottlow J, Nyman S, Lindhe J, Karring T, Wennström J. New attachment formation in the human periodontium by guided tissue regeneration. Case reports. J Clin Periodontol 1986;13:604–616.

62. Sculean A, Donos N, Chiantella GC, Windisch P, Reich E, Brecx M. GTR with bioresorbable membranes in the treatment of intrabony defects: A clinical and histologic study. Int J Periodontics Restorative Dent 1999;19:501–509.

63. Sculean A, Donos N, Windisch P, et al. Healing of human intrabony defects following treatment with enamel matrix proteins or guided tissue regeneration. J Periodontal Res 1999;34:310–322.

64. Abitbol T, Santi E, Scherer W. Use of a resin-ionomer in guided tissue regeneration: Case reports. Am J Dent 1995;8:267–269.

65. Cortellini P, Prato GP. Guided tissue regeneration with a rubber dam: A five-case report. Int J Periodontics Restorative Dent 1994;14:8–15.

66. Paolantonio M, D'Archivio D, Di Placido G, et al. Expanded polytetrafluoroethylene and dental rubber dam barrier membranes in the treatment of periodontal intrabony defects. A comparative clinical trial. J Clin Periodontol 1998;25:920–928.

67. Gottlow J. Guided tissue regeneration using bioresorbable and non-resorbable devices: Initial healing and long-term results. J Periodontol 1993;64(suppl 11):1157–1165.

68. Tatakis DN, Promsudthi A, Wikesjö UM. Devices for periodontal regeneration. Periodontol 2000 1999;19:59–73.

69. Trombelli L, Lee MB, Promsudthi A, Guglielmoni PG, Wikesjö UM. Periodontal repair in dogs: Histologic observations of guided tissue regeneration with a prostaglandin E1 analog/methacrylate composite. J Clin Periodontol 1999;26:381–387.

70. Becker W, Becker BE, Prichard JF, Caffesse R, Rosenberg E, Gian-Grasso J. Root isolation for new attachment procedures. A surgical and suturing method: Three case reports. J Periodontol 1987;58:819–826.

71. Stahl SS, Froum S, Tarnow D. Human histologic responses to guided tissue regenerative techniques in intrabony lesions. Case reports on 9 sites. J Clin Periodontol 1990;17:191–198.

72. Stahl SS, Froum SJ. Healing of human suprabony lesions treated with guided tissue regeneration and coronally anchored flaps. Case reports. J Clin Periodontol 1991;18:69–74.

73. Pihlstrom BL, McHugh RB, Oliphant TH, Ortiz-Campos C. Comparison of surgical and nonsurgical treatment of periodontal disease. A review of current studies and additional results after 6 1/2 years. J Clin Periodontol 1983;10:524–541.

74. Cortellini P, Pini Prato G, Tonetti MS. Interproximal free gingival grafts after membrane removal in guided tissue regeneration treatment of intrabony defects. A randomized controlled clinical trial. J Periodontol 1995;66:488–493.

75. Tonetti MS, Pini-Prato G, Cortellini P. Periodontal regeneration of human intrabony defects. IV. Determinants of healing response. J Periodontol 1993;64:934–940.

76. Galgut PN. Oxidized cellulose mesh used as a biodegradable barrier membrane in the technique of guided tissue regeneration. A case report. J Periodontol 1990;61:766–768.

77. Galgut PN. A technique for treatment of extensive periodontal defects: A case study. J Oral Rehabil 1994;21:27–32.

78. Sottosanti J. Calcium sulfate: A biodegradable and biocompatible barrier for guided tissue regeneration. Compendium 1992;13:226–228, 230, 232–224.

79. Warrer K, Karring T, Nyman S, Gogolewski S. Guided tissue regeneration using biodegradable membranes of polylactic acid or polyurethane. J Clin Periodontol 1992;19:633–640.

80. Camelo M, Nevins ML, Schenk RK, et al. Clinical, radiographic, and histologic evaluation of human periodontal defects treated with Bio Oss and Bio Gide. Int J Periodontics Restorative Dent 1998;18:321–331.

81. Garrett S, Loos B, Chamberlain D, Egelberg J. Treatment of intraosseous periodontal defects with a combined adjunctive therapy of citric acid conditioning, bone grafting, and placement of collagenous membranes. J Clin Periodontol 1988;15:383–389.

82. Mellonig JT. Human histologic evaluation of a bovine-derived bone xenograft in the treatment of periodontal osseous defects. Int J Periodontics Restorative Dent 2000;20:19–29.

83. Scott TA, Towle HJ, Assad DA, Nicoll BK. Comparison of bioabsorbable laminar bone membrane and non-resorbable ePTFE membrane in mandibular furcations. J Periodontol 1997;68:679–686.

84. Tatakis DN, Trombelli L. Adverse effects associated with a bioabsorbable guided tissue regeneration device in the treatment of human gingival recession defects. A clinicopathologic case report. J Periodontol 1999;70:542–547.

85. Stavropoulos A. Guided Tissue Regeneration in Combination with Deproteinized Bovine Bone and Gentamicin [thesis]. Aarhus, Denmark: Aarhus Univeristy, 2002.

86. Greenstein G, Caton JG. Biodegradable barriers and guided tissue regeneration. Periodontol 2000 1993;1:36–45.

87. Cortellini P, Tonetti MS. Radiographic defect angle influences the outcome of GTR therapy in intrabony defects [abstract 2208]. J Dent Res 1999;78(suppl 1):381.

88. Blumenthal NM. The use of collagen membranes to guide regeneration of new connective tissue attachment in dogs. J Periodontol 1988;59:830–836.

89. Caffesse RG, Nasjleti CE, Morrison EC, Sanchez R. Guided tissue regeneration: Comparison of bioabsorbable and non-bioabsorbable membranes. Histologic and histometric study in dogs. J Periodontol 1994;65:583–591.

90. Cirelli JA, Marcantonio E Jr, Adriana R, et al. Evaluation of anionic collagen membranes in the treatment of class II furcation lesions: An histometric analysis in dogs. Biomaterials 1997;18:1227–1234.

91. Fleisher N, de Waal H, Bloom A. Regeneration of lost attachment apparatus in the dog using Vicryl absorbable mesh (polyglactin 910). Int J Periodontics Restorative Dent 1988;8:44–55.

92. Gottlow J, Laurell L, Lundgren D, et al. Periodontal tissue response to a new bioresorbable guided tissue regeneration device: A longitudinal study in monkeys. Int J Periodontics Restorative Dent 1994;14:436–449.

93. Magnusson I, Batich C, Collins BR. New attachment formation following controlled tissue regeneration using biodegradable membranes. J Periodontol 1988;59:1–6.

94. Chaves ES, Geurs NC, Reddy MS, Jeffcoat MK. Clinical and radiographic digital imaging evaluation of a bioresorbable membrane in the treatment of periodontal bone defects. Int J Periodontics Restorative Dent 1996;16:443–453.

95. Murphy KG, Gunsolley JC. Guided tissue regeneration for the treatment of periodontal intrabony and furcation defects. A systematic review. Ann Periodontol 2003;8:266–302.

96. Stavropoulos A, Karring T. Long-term stability of periodontal conditions achieved following guided tissue regeneration with bioresorbable membranes: Case series results after 6-7 years. J Clin Periodontol 2004;31:939–944.

97. Christgau M, Schmalz G, Wenzel A, Hiller KA. Periodontal regeneration of intrabony defects with resorbable and non-resorbable membranes: 30-month results. J Clin Periodontol 1997;24:17–27.

98. Sculean A, Donos N, Miliauskaite A, Arweiler N, Brecx M. Treatment of intrabony defects with enamel matrix proteins or bioabsorbable membranes. A 4-year follow-up split-mouth study. J Periodontol 2001;72:1695–1701.

99. Cortellini P, Paolo G, Prato P, Tonetti MS. Long-term stability of clinical attachment following guided tissue regeneration and conventional therapy. J Clin Periodontol 1996;23:106–111.

100. Cortellini P, Pini-Prato G, Tonetti M. Periodontal regeneration of human infrabony defects (V). Effect of oral hygiene on long-term stability. J Clin Periodontol 1994;21:606–610.

101. Cortellini P, Stalpers G, Pini Prato G, Tonetti MS. Long-term clinical outcomes of abutments treated with guided tissue regeneration. J Prosthet Dent 1999;81:305–311.

102. Dragoo MR, Sullivan HC. A clinical and histological evaluation of autogenous iliac bone grafts in humans. II. External root resorption. J Periodontol 1973;44:614–625.

103. Dragoo MR, Sullivan HC. A clinical and histological evaluation of autogenous iliac bone grafts in humans. I. Wound healing 2 to 8 months. J Periodontol 1973;44:599–613.

104. Guida L, Annunziata M, Belardo S, Farina R, Scabbia A, Trombelli L. Effect of autogenous cortical bone particulate in conjunction with enamel matrix derivative in the treatment of periodontal intraosseous defects. J Periodontol 2007;78:231–238.

105. Trombelli L, Annunziata M, Belardo S, Farina R, Scabbia A, Guida L. Autogenous bone graft in conjunction with enamel matrix derivative in the treatment of deep periodontal intra-osseous defects: A report of 13 consecutively treated patients. J Clin Periodontol 2006;33:69–75.

106. Sculean A, Nikolidakis D, Nikou G, Ivanovic A, Chapple IL, Stavropoulos A. Biomaterials for promoting periodontal regeneration in human intrabony defects: A systematic review. Periodontol 2000 2015;68:182–216.

107. Hiatt WH, Schallhorn RG, Aaronian AJ. The induction of new bone and cementum formation. IV. Microscopic examination of the periodontium following human bone and marrow allograft, autograft and nongraft periodontal regenerative procedures. J Periodontol 1978;49:495–512.

108. Nabers CL, Reed OM, Hamner JE 3rd. Gross and histologic evaluation of an autogenous bone graft 57 months postoperatively. J Periodontol 1972;43:702–704.

109. Ross SE, Cohen DW. The fate of a free osseous tissue autograft. A clinical and histologic case report. Periodontics 1968;6:145–151.

110. Stahl SS, Froum SJ, Kushner L. Healing responses of human intraosseous lesions following the use of debridement, grafting and citric acid root treatment. II. Clinical and histologic observations: One year postsurgery. J Periodontol 1983;54:325–338.

111. Froum SJ, Kushner L, Stahl SS. Healing responses of human intraosseous lesions following the use of debridement, grafting and citric acid root treatment. I. Clinical and histologic observations six months postsurgery. J Periodontol 1983;54:67–76.

112. Hawley CE, Miller J. A histologic examination of a free osseous autograft. Case report. J Periodontol 1975;46:289–293.

113. Listgarten MA, Rosenberg MM. Histological study of repair following new attachment procedures in human periodontal lesions. J Periodontol 1979;50:333–344.

114. Evans RL. A clinical and histologic observation of the healing of an intrabony lesion. Int J Periodontics Restorative Dent 1981;1:20–25.

115. Moskow BS, Karsh F, Stein SD. Histological assessment of autogenous bone graft. A case report and critical evaluation. J Periodontol 1979;50:291–300.

116. Zubery Y, Kozlovsky A, Tal H. Histologic assessment of a contiguous autogenous transplant in a human intrabony defect. A case report. J Periodontol 1993;64:66–71.

117. Goldberg VM, Stevenson S. Natural history of autografts and allografts. Clin Orthop Relat Res 1987;225:7–16.

118. Dragoo MR, Kaldahl WB. Clinical and histological evaluation of alloplasts and allografts in regenerative periodontal surgery in humans. Int J Periodontics Restorative Dent 1983;3:8–29.

119. Altiere ET, Reeve CM, Sheridan PJ. Lyophilized bone allografts in periodontal intraosseous defects. J Periodontol 1979;50:510–519.

120. Mellonig JT, Bowers GM, Bailey RC. Comparison of bone graft materials. Part I. New bone formation with autografts and allografts determined by Strontium-85. J Periodontol 1981;52:291–296.

121. Urist MR, Strates BS. Bone formation in implants of partially and wholly demineralized bone matrix. Including observations on acetone-fixed intra and extracellular proteins. Clin Orthop Relat Res 1970;71:271–278.

122. Caplanis N, Lee MB, Zimmerman GJ, Selvig KA, Wikesjö UM. Effect of allogeneic freeze-dried demineralized bone matrix on regeneration of alveolar bone and periodontal attachment in dogs. J Clin Periodontol 1998;25:801–806.

123. Sonis ST, Williams RC, Jeffcoat MK, Black R, Shklar G. Healing of spontaneous periodontal defects in dogs treated with xenogeneic demineralized bone. J Periodontol 1985;56:470–479.

124. Bowers GM, Chadroff B, Carnevale R, et al. Histologic evaluation of new attachment apparatus formation in humans. Part II. J Periodontol 1989;60:675–682.

125. Bowers GM, Chadroff B, Carnevale R, et al. Histologic evaluation of new attachment apparatus formation in humans. Part III. J Periodontol 1989;60:683–693.

126. Bowers G, Felton F, Middleton C, et al. Histologic comparison of regeneration in human intrabony defects when osteogenin is combined with demineralized freeze-dried bone allograft and with purified bovine collagen. J Periodontol 1991;62:690–702.

127. Mellonig JT. Histologic and clinical evaluation of an allogeneic bone matrix for the treatment of periodontal osseous defects. Int J Periodontics Restorative Dent 2006;26:561–569.

128. Koylass JM, Valderrama P, Mellonig JT. Histologic evaluation of an allogeneic mineralized bone matrix in the treatment of periodontal osseous defects. Int J Periodontics Restorative Dent 2012;32:405–411.

129. Froum SJ. Human histologic evaluation of HTR polymer and freeze-dried bone allograft. A case report. J Clin Periodontol 1996;23:615–620.

130. Flemmig TF, Ehmke B, Bolz K, et al. Long-term maintenance of alveolar bone gain after implantation of auto-lyzed, antigen-extracted, allogenic bone in periodontal intraosseous defects. J Periodontol 1998;69:47–53.

131. Pearson GE, Rosen S, Deporter DA. Preliminary observations on the usefulness of a decalcified, freeze-dried cancellous bone allograft material in periodontal surgery. J Periodontol 1981;52:55–59.

132. Sculean A, Windisch P, Keglevich T, Chiantella GC, Gera I, Donos N. Clinical and histologic evaluation of human intrabony defects treated with an enamel matrix protein derivative combined with a bovine-derived xenograft. Int J Periodontics Restorative Dent 2003;23:47–55.

133. Nevins ML, Camelo M, Lynch SE, Schenk RK, Nevins M. Evaluation of periodontal regeneration following grafting intrabony defects with Bio-Oss collagen: A human histologic report. Int J Periodontics Restorative Dent 2003;23:9–17.

134. Richardson CR, Mellonig JT, Brunsvold MA, McDonnell HT, Cochran DL. Clinical evaluation of Bio-Oss: A bovine-derived xenograft for the treatment of periodontal osseous defects in humans. J Clin Periodontol 1999;26:421–428.

135. Yukna RA. Clinical evaluation of coralline calcium carbonate as a bone replacement graft material in human periodontal osseous defects. J Periodontol 1994;65:177–185.

136. Yukna RA, Yukna CN. A 5-year follow-up of 16 patients treated with coralline calcium carbonate (BIOCORAL) bone replacement grafts in infrabony defects. J Clin Periodontol 1998;25:1036–1040.

137. Barnett JD, Mellonig JT, Gray JL, Towle HJ. Comparison of freeze-dried bone allograft and porous hydroxylap-atite in human periodontal defects. J Periodontol 1989;60:231–237.

138. Bowen JA, Mellonig JT, Gray JL, Towle HT. Comparison of decalcified freeze-dried bone allograft and porous particulate hydroxyapatite in human periodontal osseous defects. J Periodontol 1989;60:647–654.

139. Carranza FA Jr, Kenney EB, Lekovic V, Talamante E, Valencia J, Dimitrijevic B. Histologic study of healing of human periodontal defects after placement of porous hydroxylapatite implants. J Periodontol 1987;58:682–688.

140. Ettel RG, Schaffer EM, Holpuch RC, Bandt CL. Porous hydroxyapatite grafts in chronic subcrestal periodontal defects in rhesus monkeys: A histological investigation. J Periodontol 1989;60:342–351.

141. West TL, Brustein DD. Freeze-dried bone and coralline implants compared in the dog. J Periodontol 1985;56:348–351.

142. Carraro JJ, Sznajder N, Alonso CA. Intraoral cancellous bone autografts in the treatment of infrabony pockets. J Clin Periodontol 1976;3:104–109.

143. Froum SJ, Kushner L, Scopp IW, Stahl SS. Human clinical and histologic responses to Durapatite implants in intraosseous lesions. Case reports. J Periodontol 1982;53:719–725.

144. Rühling A, Plagmann HC. Hydroxylapatit und bioglas in parodontalen knochentaschen- klinisch-röntgenolo-gische versus histologische befunde. Parodontologie 2001;13:261–271.

145. Sibilla P, Sereni A, Aguiari G, et al. Effects of a hydroxyapatite-based biomaterial on gene expression in osteo-blast-like cells. J Dent Res 2006;85:354–358.

146. Trombelli L, Penolazzi L, Torreggiani E, et al. Effect of hydroxyapatite-based biomaterials on human osteoblast phenotype. Minerva Stomatol 2010;59:103–115.

147. Manfrini M, Mazzoni E, Barbanti-Brodano G, et al. Osteoconductivity of complex biomaterials assayed by fluorescent-engineered osteoblast-like cells. Cell Biochem Biophys 2015;71:1509–1515.

148. Barney VC, Levin MP, Adams DF. Bioceramic implants in surgical periodontal defects. A comparison study. J Periodontol 1986;57:764–770.

149. Horváth A, Stavropoulos A, Windisch P, Lukács L, Gera I, Sculean A. Histological evaluation of human intra-bony periodontal defects treated with an unsintered nanocrystalline hydroxyapatite paste. Clin Oral Investig 2013;17:423–430.

150. Wilson J, Low SB. Bioactive ceramics for periodontal treatment: Comparative studies in the Patus monkey. J Appl Biomater 1992;3:123–129.

151. Galgut PN, Waite IM, Brookshaw JD, Kingston CP. A 4-year controlled clinical study into the use of a ceramic hydroxylapatite implant material for the treatment of periodontal bone defects. J Clin Periodontol 1992;19:570–577.

152. Meffert RM, Thomas JR, Hamilton KM, Brownstein CN. Hydroxylapatite as an alloplastic graft in the treatment of human periodontal osseous defects. J Periodontol 1985;56:63–73.

153. Yukna RA, Harrison BG, Caudill RF, Evans GH, Mayer ET, Miller S. Evaluation of durapatite ceramic as an al-loplastic implant in periodontal osseous defects. II. Twelve month reentry results. J Periodontol 1985;56:540–547.

154. Trombelli L, Simonelli A, Pramstraller M, Wikesjö UM, Farina R. Single flap approach with and without guided tissue regeneration and a hydroxyapatite biomaterial in the management of intraosseous periodontal defects. J Periodontol 2010;81:1256–1263.

155. Stein JM, Fickl S, Yekta SS, Hoischen U, Ocklenburg C, Smeets R. Clinical evaluation of a biphasic calcium composite grafting material in the treatment of human periodontal intrabony defects: A 12-month randomized controlled clinical trial. J Periodontol 2009;80:1774–1782.

156. Scabbia A, Trombelli L. A comparative study on the use of a HA/collagen/chondroitin sulphate biomaterial (Biostite) and a bovine-derived HA xenograft (Bio-Oss) in the treatment of deep intra-osseous defects. J Clin Periodontol 2004;31:348–55.

157. Trombelli L, Heitz-Mayfield LJ, Needleman I, Moles D, Scabbia A. A systematic review of graft materials and biological agents for periodontal intraosseous defects. J Clin Periodontol 2002;29(suppl 3):117–135.

158. Baldock WT, Hutchens LH Jr, McFall WT Jr, Simpson DM. An evaluation of tricalcium phosphate implants in human periodontal osseous defects of two patients. J Periodontol 1985;56:1–7.

159. Snyder AJ, Levin MP, Cutright DE. Alloplastic implants of tricalcium phosphate ceramic in human periodontal osseous defects. J Periodontol 1984;55:273–277.

160. Strub JR, Gaberthüel TW, Firestone AR. Comparison of tricalcium phosphate and frozen allogenic bone implants in man. J Periodontol 1979;50:624–629.

161. Levin MP, Getter L, Adrian J, Cutright DE. Healing of periodontal defects with ceramic implants. J Clin Periodontol 1974;1:197–205.

162. Stavropoulos A, Windisch P, Szendröi-Kiss D, Peter R, Gera I, Sculean A. Clinical and histologic evaluation of granular Beta-tricalcium phosphate for the treatment of human intrabony periodontal defects: A report on five cases. J Periodontol 2010;81:325–334.

163. Plotzke AE, Barbosa S, Nasjleti CE, Morrison EC, Caffesse RG. Histologic and histometric responses to polymeric composite grafts. J Periodontol 1993;64:343–348.

164. Stahl SS, Froum SJ, Tarnow D. Human clinical and histologic responses to the placement of HTR polymer particles in 11 intrabony lesions. J Periodontol 1990;61:269–274.

165. Shahmiri S, Singh IJ, Stahl SS. Clinical response to the use of the HTR polymer implant in human intrabony lesions. Int J Periodontics Restorative Dent 1992;12:294–299.

166. Yukna RA. HTR polymer grafts in human periodontal osseous defects. I. 6-month clinical results. J Periodontol 1990;61:633–642.

167. Minenna L, Herrero F, Sanz M, Trombelli L. Adjunctive effect of a polylactide/polyglycolide copolymer in the treatment of deep periodontal intra-osseous defects: A randomized clinical trial. J Clin Periodontol 2005;32:456–461.

168. Karatzas S, Zavras A, Greenspan D, Amar S. Histologic observations of periodontal wound healing after treatment with PerioGlas in nonhuman primates. Int J Periodontics Restorative Dent 1999;19:489–499.

169. Nevins ML, Camelo M, Nevins M, et al. Human histologic evaluation of bioactive ceramic in the treatment of periodontal osseous defects. Int J Periodontics Restorative Dent 2000;20:458–467.

170. Sculean A, Windisch P, Keglevich T, Gera I. Clinical and histologic evaluation of an enamel matrix protein derivative combined with a bioactive glass for the treatment of intrabony periodontal defects in humans. Int J Periodontics Restorative Dent 2005;25:139–147.

171. Ong MM, Eber RM, Korsnes MI, et al. Evaluation of a bioactive glass alloplast in treating periodontal intrabony defects. J Periodontol 1998;69:1346–1354.

172. Zamet JS, Darbar UR, Griffiths GS, et al. Particulate bioglass as a grafting material in the treatment of periodontal intrabony defects. J Clin Periodontol 1997;24:410–418.

173. Slavkin HC. Towards a cellular and molecular understanding of periodontics. Cementogenesis revisited. J Periodontol 1976;47:249–255.

174. Slavkin HC, Boyde A. Cementum: An epithelial secretory product? J Dent Res 1975;53:157.

175. Hammarström L. Enamel matrix, cementum development and regeneration. J Clin Periodontol 1997;24:658–668.

176. Brookes SJ, Robinson C, Kirkham J, Bonass WA. Biochemistry and molecular biology of amelogenin proteins of developing dental enamel. Arch Oral Biol 1995;40:1–14.

177. Sire JY, Delgado S, Fromentin D, Girondot M. Amelogenin: Lessons from evolution. Arch Oral Biol 2005;50:205–212.

178. Bartlett JD, Ganss B, Goldberg M, et al. 3. Protein-protein interactions of the developing enamel matrix. Curr Top Dev Biol 2006;74:57–115.

179. Simmer JP. Alternative splicing of amelogenins. Connect Tissue Res 1995;32:131–136.

180. Froum S, Weinberg M, Novak J, et al. A multicenter study evaluating the sensitization potential of enamel matrix derivative after treatment of two infrabony defects. J Periodontol 2004;75:1001–1008.

181. Gestrelius S, Andersson C, Johansson AC, et al. Formulation of enamel matrix derivative for surface coating. Kinetics and cell colonization. J Clin Periodontol 1997;24:678–684.

182. Gestrelius S, Andersson C, Lidström D, Hammarström L, Somerman M. In vitro studies on periodontal ligament cells and enamel matrix derivative. J Clin Periodontol 1997;24:685–692.

183. Heijl L. Periodontal regeneration with enamel matrix derivative in one human experimental defect. A case report. J Clin Periodontol 1997;24:693–696.

184. Heijl L, Heden G, Svärdström G, Ostgren A. Enamel matrix derivative (EMDOGAIN) in the treatment of intrabony periodontal defects. J Clin Periodontol 1997;24:705–714.

185. Miron RJ, Sculean A, Cochran DL, et al. Twenty years of enamel matrix derivative: The past, the present and the future. J Clin Periodontol 2016;43:668–683.

186. Sculean A, Windisch P, Keglevich T, Fabi B, Lundgren E, Lyngstadaas PS. Presence of an enamel matrix protein derivative on human teeth following periodontal surgery. Clin Oral Investig 2002;6:183–187.

187. Trombelli L, Farina R. Clinical outcomes with bioactive agents alone or in combination with grafting or guided tissue regeneration. J Clin Periodontol 2008;35:117–135.

188. Lyngstadaas SP, Lundberg E, Ekdahl H, Andersson C, Gestrelius S. Autocrine growth factors in human periodontal ligament cells cultured on enamel matrix derivative. J Clin Periodontol 2001;28:181–188.

189. Okubo K, Kobayashi M, Takiguchi T, et al. Participation of endogenous IGF-I and TGF-beta 1 with enamel matrix derivative-stimulated cell growth in human periodontal ligament cells. J Periodontal Res 2003;38:1–9.

190. Palioto DB, Coletta RD, Graner E, Joly JC, de Lima AF. The influence of enamel matrix derivative associated with insulin-like growth factor-I on periodontal ligament fibroblasts. J Periodontol 2004;75:498–504.

191. Kawase T, Okuda K, Momose M, Kato Y, Yoshie H, Burns DM. Enamel matrix derivative (EMDOGAIN) rapidly stimulates phosphorylation of the MAP kinase family and nuclear accumulation of smad2 in both oral epithelial and fibroblastic human cells. J Periodontal Res 2001;36:367–376.

192. Kawase T, Okuda K, Yoshie H, Burns DM. Anti-TGF-beta antibody blocks enamel matrix derivative-induced upregulation of p21WAF1/cip1 and prevents its inhibition of human oral epithelial cell proliferation. J Periodontal Res 2002;37:255–262.

193. Suzuki S, Nagano T, Yamakoshi Y, et al. Enamel matrix derivative gel stimulates signal transduction of BMP and TGF-{beta}. J Dent Res 2005;84:510–514.

194. Maycock J, Wood SR, Brookes SJ, Shore RC, Robinson C, Kirkham J. Characterization of a porcine amelogenin preparation, EMDOGAIN, a biological treatment for periodontal disease. Connect Tissue Res 2002;43:472–476.

195. Keila S, Nemcovsky CE, Moses O, Artzi Z, Weinreb M. In vitro effects of enamel matrix proteins on rat bone marrow cells and gingival fibroblasts. J Dent Res 2004;83:134–138.

196. Haase HR, Bartold PM. Enamel matrix derivative induces matrix synthesis by cultured human periodontal fibroblast cells. J Periodontol 2001;72:341–348.

197. Hoang AM, Oates TW, Cochran DL. In vitro wound healing responses to enamel matrix derivative. J Periodontol 2000;71:1270–1277.

198. Cattaneo V, Rota C, Silvestri M, et al. Effect of enamel matrix derivative on human periodontal fibroblasts: Proliferation, morphology and root surface colonization. An in vitro study. J Periodontal Res 2003;38:568–574.

199. Davenport DR, Mailhot JM, Wataha JC, Billman MA, Sharawy MM, Shrout MK. Effects of enamel matrix protein application on the viability, proliferation, and attachment of human periodontal ligament fibroblasts to diseased root surfaces in vitro. J Clin Periodontol 2003;30:125–131.

200. van der Pauw MT, Everts V, Beertsen W. Expression of integrins by human periodontal ligament and gingival fibroblasts and their involvement in fibroblast adhesion to enamel matrix-derived proteins. J Periodontal Res 2002;37:317–323.

201. Kawase T, Okuda K, Yoshie H, Burns DM. Cytostatic action of enamel matrix derivative (EMDOGAIN) on human oral squamous cell carcinoma-derived SCC25 epithelial cells. J Periodontal Res 2000;35:291–300.

202. Boyan BD, Weesner TC, Lohmann CH, et al. Porcine fetal enamel matrix derivative enhances bone formation induced by demineralized freeze dried bone allograft in vivo. J Periodontol 2000;71:1278–1286.

203. Parkar MH, Tonetti M. Gene expression profiles of periodontal ligament cells treated with enamel matrix proteins in vitro: Analysis using cDNA arrays. J Periodontol 2004;75:1539–1546.

204. Mirastschijski U, Konrad D, Lundberg E, Lyngstadaas SP, Jorgensen LN, Agren MS. Effects of a topical enamel matrix derivative on skin wound healing. Wound Repair Regen 2004;12:100–108.

205. Yuan K, Chen CL, Lin MT. Enamel matrix derivative exhibits angiogenic effect in vitro and in a murine model. J Clin Periodontol 2003;30:732–738.

206. Sculean A, Auschill TM, Donos N, Brecx M, Arweiler NB. Effect of an enamel matrix protein derivative (Emdogain) on ex vivo dental plaque vitality. J Clin Periodontol 2001;28:1074–1078.

207. Arweiler NB, Auschill TM, Donos N, Sculean A. Antibacterial effect of an enamel matrix protein derivative on in vivo dental biofilm vitality. Clin Oral Investig 2002;6:205–209.

208. Newman SA, Coscia SA, Jotwani R, Iacono VJ, Cutler CW. Effects of enamel matrix derivative on *Porphyromonas gingivalis*. J Periodontol 2003;74:1191–1195.

209. Spahr L, Villeneuve JP, Tran HK, Pomier-Layrargues G. Furosemide-induced natriuresis as a test to identify cirrhotic patients with refractory ascites. Hepatology 2001;33:28–31.

210. Inaba H, Kawai S, Nakayama K, Okahashi N, Amano A. Effect of enamel matrix derivative on periodontal ligament cells in vitro is diminished by *Porphyromonas gingivalis*. J Periodontol 2004;75:858–865.

211. Hammarström L, Heijl L, Gestrelius S. Periodontal regeneration in a buccal dehiscence model in monkeys after application of enamel matrix proteins. J Clin Periodontol 1997;24:669–677.

212. Yukna RA, Mellonig JT. Histologic evaluation of periodontal healing in humans following regenerative therapy with enamel matrix derivative. A 10-case series. J Periodontol 2000;71:752–759.

213. Sculean A, Donos N, Reich E, Karring T, Brecx M. Regeneration of oxytalan fibres in different types of periodontal defects: A histological study in monkeys. J Periodontal Res 1998;33:453–459.

214. Windisch P, Sculean A, Klein F, et al. Comparison of clinical, radiographic, and histometric measurements following treatment with guided tissue regeneration or enamel matrix proteins in human periodontal defects. J Periodontol 2002;73:409–417.

215. Sculean A, Chiantella GC, Windisch P, Donos N. Clinical and histologic evaluation of human intrabony defects treated with an enamel matrix protein derivative (Emdogain). Int J Periodontics Restorative Dent 2000;20:374–381.

216. Sculean A, Berakdar M, Windisch P, Remberger K, Donos N, Brecx M. Immunohistochemical investigation on the pattern of vimentin expression in regenerated and intact monkey and human periodontal ligament. Arch Oral Biol 2003;48:77–86.

217. Bosshardt DD, Sculean A, Donos N, Lang NP. Pattern of mineralization after regenerative periodontal therapy with enamel matrix proteins. Eur J Oral Sci 2006;1(suppl 114):225–231; discussion 254–256, 381–382.

218. Bosshardt DD, Sculean A, Windisch P, Pjetursson BE, Lang NP. Effects of enamel matrix proteins on tissue formation along the roots of human teeth. J Periodontal Res 2005;40:158–167.

219. Sculean A, Windisch P, Keglevich T, Gera I. Histologic evaluation of human intrabony defects following non-surgical periodontal therapy with and without application of an enamel matrix protein derivative. J Periodontol 2003;74:153–160.

220. St George G, Darbar U, Thomas G. Inflammatory external root resorption following surgical treatment for intra-bony defects: A report of two cases involving Emdogain and a review of the literature. J Clin Periodontol 2006;33:449–454.

221. Sculean A, Donos N, Brecx M, Karring T, Reich E. Healing of fenestration-type defects following treatment with guided tissue regeneration or enamel matrix proteins. An experimental study in monkeys. Clin Oral Investig 2000;4:50–56.

222. Donos N, Sculean A, Glavind L, Reich E, Karring T. Wound healing of degree III furcation involvements following guided tissue regeneration and/or Emdogain. A histologic study. J Clin Periodontol 2003;30:1061–1068.

223. Regazzini PF, Novaes AB Jr, de Oliveira PT, et al. Comparative study of enamel matrix derivative with or without GTR in the treatment of class II furcation lesions in dogs. Int J Periodontics Restorative Dent 2004;24:476–487.

224. Stavropoulos A, Wikesjö, U. Periodontal tissue engineering: Focus on growth factors. In: Sculean A (ed). Periodontal Regenerative Therapy. London: Quintessence, 2010:193–214.

225. Rosenkranz S, Kazlauskas A. Evidence for distinct signaling properties and biological responses induced by the PDGF receptor alpha and beta subtypes. Growth Factors 1999;16:201–216.

226. Terranova VP, Wikesjö UM. Extracellular matrices and polypeptide growth factors as mediators of functions of cells of the periodontium. A review. J Periodontol 1987;58:371–380.

227. Anusaksathien O, Giannobile WV. Growth factor delivery to re-engineer periodontal tissues. Curr Pharm Biotechnol 2002;3:129–139.

228. King GN, Cochran DL. Factors that modulate the effects of bone morphogenetic protein-induced periodontal regeneration: A critical review. J Periodontol 2002;73:925–936.

229. von Bubnoff A, Cho KW. Intracellular BMP signaling regulation in vertebrates: Pathway or network? Dev Biol 2001;239:1–14.

230. Ross R, Raines E, Bowen-Pope D. Growth factors from platelets, monocytes, and endothelium: Their role in cell proliferation. Ann N Y Acad Sci 1982;397:18–24.

231. Ross R, Raines EW, Bowen-Pope DF. The biology of platelet-derived growth factor. Cell 1986;46:155–169.

232. Bergsten E, Uutela M, Li X, et al. PDGF-D is a specific, protease-activated ligand for the PDGF beta-receptor. Nat Cell Biol 2001;3:512–516.

233. Uutela M, Laurén J, Bergsten E, et al. Chromosomal location, exon structure, and vascular expression patterns of the human PDGFC and PDGFD genes. Circulation 2001;103:2242–2247.

234. Dennison DK, Vallone DR, Pinero GJ, Rittman B, Caffesse RG. Differential effect of TGF-beta 1 and PDGF on proliferation of periodontal ligament cells and gingival fibroblasts. J Periodontol 1994;65:641–648.

235. Matsuda N, Lin WL, Kumar NM, Cho MI, Genco RJ. Mitogenic, chemotactic, and synthetic responses of rat periodontal ligament fibroblastic cells to polypeptide growth factors in vitro. J Periodontol 1992;63:515–525.

236. Canalis E. Effect of platelet-derived growth factor on DNA and protein synthesis in cultured rat calvaria. Metabolism 1981;30:970–975.

237. Hock JM, Canalis E. Platelet-derived growth factor enhances bone cell replication, but not differentiated function of osteoblasts. Endocrinology 1994;134:1423–1428.

238. Giannobile WV, Whitson SW, Lynch SE. Non-coordinate control of bone formation displayed by growth factor combinations with IGF-I. J Dent Res 1997;76:1569–1578.

239. Hsieh SC, Graves DT. Pulse application of platelet-derived growth factor enhances formation of a mineralizing matrix while continuous application is inhibitory. J Cell Biochem 1998;69:169–180.

240. Zaman KU, Sugaya T, Kato H. Effect of recombinant human platelet-derived growth factor-BB and bone morphogenetic protein-2 application to demineralized dentin on early periodontal ligament cell response. J Periodontal Res 1999;34:244–250.

241. Saygin NE, Tokiyasu Y, Giannobile WV, Somerman MJ. Growth factors regulate expression of mineral associated genes in cementoblasts. J Periodontol 2000;71:1591–1600.

242. Wang HL, Pappert TD, Castelli WA, Chiego DJ Jr, Shyr Y, Smith BA. The effect of platelet-derived growth factor on the cellular response of the periodontium: An autoradiographic study on dogs. J Periodontol 1994;65:429–436.

243. Park JB, Matsuura M, Han KY, et al. Periodontal regeneration in class III furcation defects of beagle dogs using guided tissue regenerative therapy with platelet-derived growth factor. J Periodontol 1995;66:462–477.

244. Giannobile WV, Hernandez RA, Finkelman RD, et al. Comparative effects of platelet-derived growth factor-BB and insulin-like growth factor-I, individually and in combination, on periodontal regeneration in *Macaca fascicularis*. J Periodontal Res 1996;31:301–312.

245. Camelo M, Nevins ML, Schenk RK, Lynch SE, Nevins M. Periodontal regeneration in human Class II furcations using purified recombinant human platelet-derived growth factor-BB (rhPDGF-BB) with bone allograft. Int J Periodontics Restorative Dent 2003;23:213–225.

246. Nevins M, Camelo M, Nevins ML, Schenk RK, Lynch SE. Periodontal regeneration in humans using recombinant human platelet-derived growth factor-BB (rhPDGF-BB) and allogenic bone. J Periodontol 2003;74:1282–1292.

247. Ridgway HK, Mellonig JT, Cochran DL. Human histologic and clinical evaluation of recombinant human platelet-derived growth factor and beta-tricalcium phosphate for the treatment of periodontal intraosseous defects. Int J Periodontics Restorative Dent 2008;28:171–179.

248. Clemmons DR. Insulin-like growth factors: Their binding proteins and growth regulation. In: Canalis E (ed). Skeletal Growth Factors. Philadelphia: Lippincott, Williams and Wilkins, 2000:79–100.

249. Nishimura F, Terranova VP. Comparative study of the chemotactic responses of periodontal ligament cells and gingival fibroblasts to polypeptide growth factors. J Dent Res 1996;75:986–992.

250. Hock JM, Centrella M, Canalis E. Insulin-like growth factor I has independent effects on bone matrix formation and cell replication. Endocrinology 1988;122:254–260.

251. Strayhorn CL, Garrett JS, Dunn RL, Benedict JJ, Somerman MJ. Growth factors regulate expression of osteoblast-associated genes. J Periodontol 1999;70:1345–1354.

252. Spencer EM, Liu CC, Si EC, Howard GA. In vivo actions of insulin-like growth factor-I (IGF-I) on bone formation and resorption in rats. Bone 1991;12:21–26.

253. Lynch SE, Williams RC, Polson AM, Reddy MS, Howell TH, Antoniades HN. Effect of insulin-like growth factor-I on periodontal regeneration. J Dent Res 1989;68:394.

254. Lynch SE, de Castilla GR, Williams RC, et al. The effects of short-term application of a combination of platelet-derived and insulin-like growth factors on periodontal wound healing. J Periodontol 1991;62:458–467.

255. Lynch SE, Williams RC, Polson AM, et al. A combination of platelet-derived and insulin-like growth factors enhances periodontal regeneration. J Clin Periodontol 1989;16:545–548.

256. Howell TH, Fiorellini JP, Paquette DW, Offenbacher S, Giannobile WV, Lynch SE. A phase I/II clinical trial to evaluate a combination of recombinant human platelet-derived growth factor BB and recombinant human insulin-like growth factor-I in patients with periodontal disease. J Periodontol 1997;68:1186–1193.

257. Ledoux D, Gannoun-Zaki L, Barritault D. Interactions of FGFs with target cells. Prog Growth Factor Res 1992;4:107–120.

258. Globus RK, Plouet J, Gospodarowicz D. Cultured bovine bone cells synthesize basic fibroblast growth factor and store it in their extracellular matrix. Endocrinology 1989;124:1539–1547.

259. Gao J, Jordan TW, Cutress TW. Immunolocalization of basic fibroblast growth factor (bFGF) in human periodontal ligament (PDL) tissue. J Periodontal Res 1996;31:260–264.

260. Murakami S, Takayama S, Ikezawa K, et al. Regeneration of periodontal tissues by basic fibroblast growth factor. J Periodontal Res 1999;34:425–430.

261. Terranova VP, Odziemiec C, Tweden KS, Spadone DP. Repopulation of dentin surfaces by periodontal ligament cells and endothelial cells. Effect of basic fibroblast growth factor. J Periodontol 1989;60:293–301.

262. Murakami S, Takayama S, Kitamura M, et al. Recombinant human basic fibroblast growth factor (bFGF) stimulates periodontal regeneration in class II furcation defects created in beagle dogs. J Periodontal Res 2003;38:97–103.

263. Takayama S, Murakami S, Shimabukuro Y, Kitamura M, Okada H. Periodontal regeneration by FGF-2 (bFGF) in primate models. J Dent Res 2001;80:2075–2079.

264. Rossa C Jr, Marcantonio E Jr, Cirelli JA, Marcantonio RA, Spolidorio LC, Fogo JC. Regeneration of Class III furcation defects with basic fibroblast growth factor (b-FGF) associated with GTR. A descriptive and histometric study in dogs. J Periodontol 2000;71:775–784.

265. Takahashi D, Odajima T, Morita M, Kawanami M, Kato H. Formation and resolution of ankylosis under application of recombinant human bone morphogenetic protein-2 (rhBMP-2) to class III furcation defects in cats. J Periodontal Res 2005;40:299–305.

266. Roberts A. Transformig growth factor-b. In: Canalis E (ed). Skeletal Growth Factors. Philadelphia: Lippincott, Williams and Wilkins, 2000.

267. Gao J, Symons AL, Bartold PM. Expression of transforming growth factor-beta receptors types II and III within various cells in the rat periodontium. J Periodontal Res 1999;34:113–122.

268. Parkar MH, Kuru L, Giouzeli M, Olsen I. Expression of growth-factor receptors in normal and regenerating human periodontal cells. Arch Oral Biol 2001;46:275–284.

269. Bonewald LF, Mundy GR. Role of transforming growth factor-beta in bone remodeling. Clin Orthop Relat Res 1990;250:261–276.

270. Hock JM, Canalis E, Centrella M. Transforming growth factor-beta stimulates bone matrix apposition and bone cell replication in cultured fetal rat calvariae. Endocrinology 1990;126:421–426.

271. Oreffo RO, Mundy GR, Seyedin SM, Bonewald LF. Activation of the bone-derived latent TGF beta complex by isolated osteoclasts. Biochem Biophys Res Commun 1989;158:817–823.

272. Mohammed S, Pack AR, Kardos TB. The effect of transforming growth factor beta one (TGF-beta 1) on wound healing, with or without barrier membranes, in a Class II furcation defect in sheep. J Periodontal Res 1998;33:335–344.

273. Tatakis DN, Wikesjö UM, Razi SS, et al. Periodontal repair in dogs: Effect of transforming growth factor-beta 1 on alveolar bone and cementum regeneration. J Clin Periodontol 2000;27:698–704.

274. Wikesjö UM, Lim WH, Razi SS, et al. Periodontal repair in dogs: A bioabsorbable calcium carbonate coral implant enhances space provision for alveolar bone regeneration in conjunction with guided tissue regeneration. J Periodontol 2003;74:957–964.

275. Wikesjö UM, Razi SS, Sigurdsson TJ, et al. Periodontal repair in dogs: Effect of recombinant human transforming growth factor-beta1 on guided tissue regeneration. J Clin Periodontol 1998;25:475–481.

276. Koo KT, Susin C, Wikesjö UM, Choi SH, Kim CK. Transforming growth factor-beta1 accelerates resorption of a calcium carbonate biomaterial in periodontal defects. J Periodontol 2007;78:723–729.

277. Urist MR. Bone: Formation by autoinduction. Science 1965;150:893–899.

278. Reddi AH. Role of morphogenetic proteins in skeletal tissue engineering and regeneration. Nat Biotechnol 1998;16:247–252.

279. Reddi AH. Bone morphogenetic proteins: From basic science to clinical applications. J Bone Joint Surg Am 2001;83-A(suppl 1):S1–S6.

280. Sena K, Morotome Y, Baba O, Terashima T, Takano Y, Ishikawa I. Gene expression of growth differentiation factors in the developing periodontium of rat molars. J Dent Res 2003;82:166–171.

281. Thomadakis G, Ramoshebi LN, Crooks J, Rueger DC, Ripamonti U. Immunolocalization of bone morphogenetic protein-2 and -3 and osteogenic protein-1 during murine tooth root morphogenesis and in other craniofacial structures. Eur J Oral Sci 1999;107:368–377.

282. Wolfman NM, Hattersley G, Cox K, et al. Ectopic induction of tendon and ligament in rats by growth and differentiation factors 5, 6, and 7, members of the TGF-beta gene family. J Clin Invest 1997;100:321–330.

283. Sigurdsson TJ, Lee MB, Kubota K, Turek TJ, Wozney JM, Wikesjö UM. Periodontal repair in dogs: Recombinant human bone morphogenetic protein-2 significantly enhances periodontal regeneration. J Periodontol 1995;66:131–138.

284. Wikesjö UM, Guglielmoni P, Promsudthi A, et al. Periodontal repair in dogs: Effect of rhBMP-2 concentration on regeneration of alveolar bone and periodontal attachment. J Clin Periodontol 1999;26:392–400.

285. Sigurdsson TJ, Nygaard L, Tatakis DN, et al. Periodontal repair in dogs: Evaluation of rhBMP-2 carriers. Int J Periodontics Restorative Dent 1996;16:524–537.

286. Wikesjö UM, Xiropaidis AV, Thomson RC, Cook AD, Selvig KA, Hardwick WR. Periodontal repair in dogs: Space-providing ePTFE devices increase rhBMP-2/ACS-induced bone formation. J Clin Periodontol 2003;30:715–725.

287. Blumenthal NM, Koh-Kunst G, Alves ME, et al. Effect of surgical implantation of recombinant human bone morphogenetic protein-2 in a bioabsorbable collagen sponge or calcium phosphate putty carrier in intrabony periodontal defects in the baboon. J Periodontol 2002;73:1494–1506.

288. King GN, King N, Cruchley AT, Wozney JM, Hughes FJ. Recombinant human bone morphogenetic protein-2 promotes wound healing in rat periodontal fenestration defects. J Dent Res 1997;76:1460–1470.

289. Ripamonti U, Heliotis M, van den Heever B, Reddi AH. Bone morphogenetic proteins induce periodontal regeneration in the baboon (*Papio ursinus*). J Periodontal Res 1994;29:439–445.

290. Huang KK, Shen C, Chiang CY, Hsieh YD, Fu E. Effects of bone morphogenetic protein-6 on periodontal wound healing in a fenestration defect of rats. J Periodontal Res 2005;40:1–10.

291. Ripamonti U, Heliotis M, Rueger DC, Sampath TK. Induction of cementogenesis by recombinant human osteogenic protein-1 (hop-1/bmp-7) in the baboon (Papio ursinus). Arch Oral Biol 1996;41:121–126.

292. Ripamonti U, Crooks J, Teare J, Petit JC, Rueger DC. Periodontal tissue regeneration by recombinant human osteogenic protein-1 in periodontally-induced furcation defects of the primate *Papio ursinus*. S Afr J Sci 2002;98:361–368.

293. Giannobile WV, Ryan S, Shih MS, Su DL, Kaplan PL, Chan TC. Recombinant human osteogenic protein-1 (OP-1) stimulates periodontal wound healing in class III furcation defects. J Periodontol 1998;69:129–137.

294. Ripamonti U, Crooks J, Petit JC, Rueger DC. Periodontal tissue regeneration by combined applications of recombinant human osteogenic protein-1 and bone morphogenetic protein-2. A pilot study in Chacma baboons (*Papio ursinus*). Eur J Oral Sci 2001;109:241–248.

295. Wikesjö UM, Sorensen RG, Kinoshita A, Jian Li X, Wozney JM. Periodontal repair in dogs: Effect of recombinant human bone morphogenetic protein-12 (rhBMP-12) on regeneration of alveolar bone and periodontal attachment. J Clin Periodontol 2004;31:662–670.

296. Kim CS, Choi SH, Cho KS, Chai JK, Wikesjö UM, Kim CK. Periodontal healing in one-wall intra-bony defects in dogs following implantation of autogenous bone or a coral-derived biomaterial. J Clin Periodontol 2005;32:583–589.

297. Kwon HR, Wikesjö UM, Jung UW et al. Periodontal regeneration following implantation of rhGDF-5 vs rhPDGF in dogs. J Dent Res 2009;(special issue):abstract 1711.

298. Stavropoulos A, Windisch P, Gera I, Capsius B, Sculean A, Wikesjö UM. A phase IIa randomized controlled clinical and histological pilot study evaluating rhGDF-5/beta-TCP for periodontal regeneration. J Clin Periodontol 2011;38:1044–1054.

299. Windisch P, Stavropoulos A, Molnár B, et al. A phase IIa randomized controlled pilot study evaluating the safety and clinical outcomes following the use of rhGDF-5/beta-TCP in regenerative periodontal therapy. Clin Oral Investig 2012;16:1181–1189.

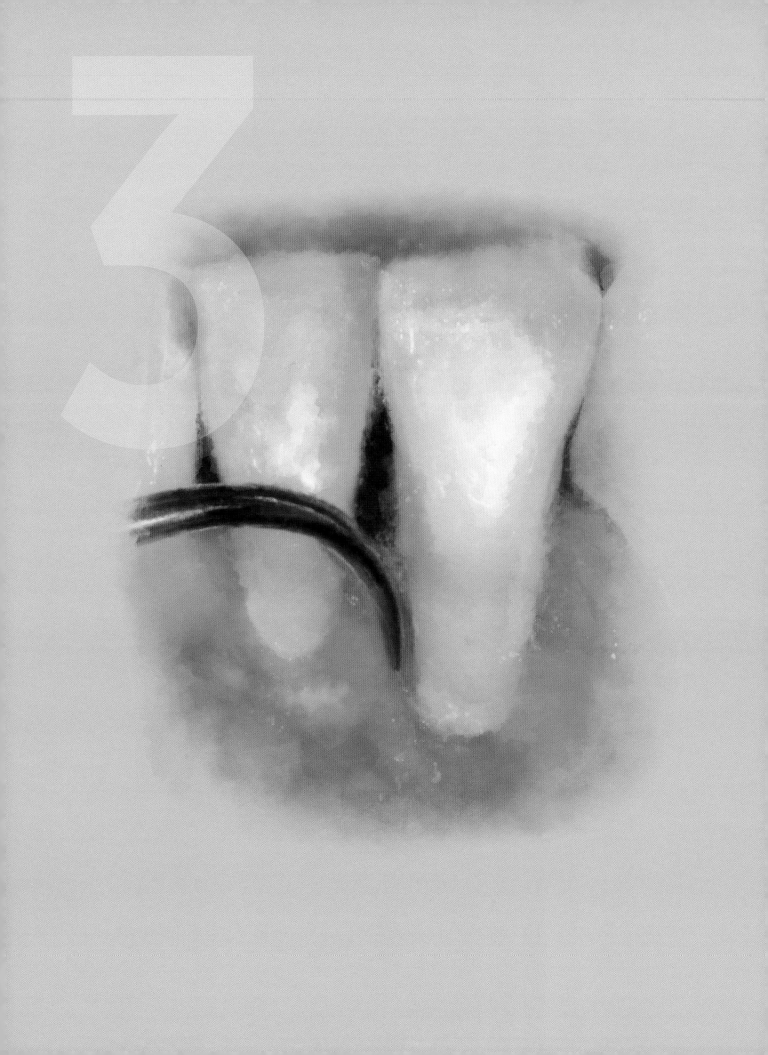

NONSURGICAL TREATMENT OF INTRAOSSEOUS DEFECTS

Mario Aimetti, MD, DDS

Giulia Maria Mariani, DDS, MSc

Federica Romano, DDS

Anna Simonelli, DDS, PhD

Leonardo Trombelli, DDS, PhD

NONSURGICAL MANAGEMENT OF PERIODONTITIS

Main goals of nonsurgical therapy

Periodontitis is a complex chronic inflammatory disease of the tissues supporting the tooth. It causes the breakdown of connective tissue attachment and alveolar bone, and if left untreated, it may lead to tooth loss.[1] The dysbiosis within the human dental plaque biofilm is the primary initiator of periodontal disease, even though the extent and severity of tissue destruction appear to be mediated by the host.[2,3] Hereditary, systemic, and environmental factors such as diabetes mellitus, connective tissue and hematologic disorders, and smoking habits have been proven to modulate the host response to the bacterial aggression.[4,5] Because it is impossible to modify the individual susceptibility to periodontal disease, biofilm control is still essential for the treatment of periodontitis[6,7] (Fig 3-1). There is increasing evidence that periodontitis also plays a significant role in general health, so treating it effectively may be paramount for both oral health and systemic health.[8]

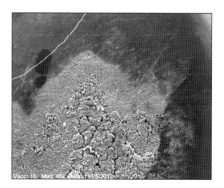

Fig 3-1 Subgingival calculus deposit on the root surface (scanning electron microscope, original magnification ×48; courtesy of Dr Agostino Scipioni).

In recent years, *appropriateness* has become a recognized element of health care system performance: Available evidence and expert opinion must demonstrate that the expected benefits outweigh the expected harms. The American Academy of Periodontology (AAP)

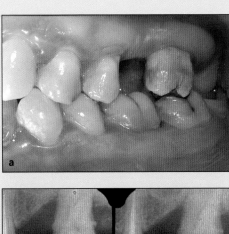
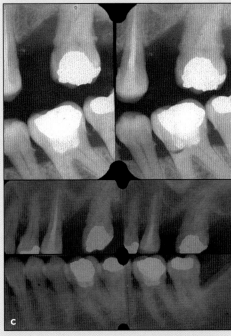
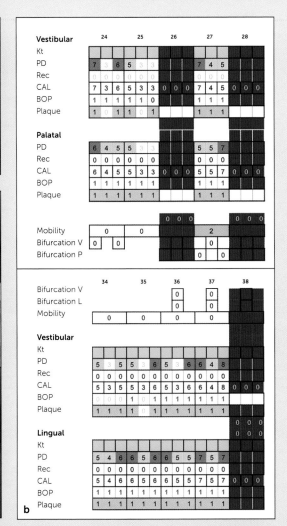

Fig 3-2 *(a to c)* Supra- and subgingival calculus in a patient with Stage III, Grade B periodontitis. Dental calculus has been considered a secondary etiologic factor in periodontitis as it provides an ideal niche for plaque retention. Abundant subgingival calculus deposits may be visible on radiographs. Periodontal examination revealed probing depths (PDs) from 4 to 8 mm, bleeding on probing (BOP) in multiple sites, and Class II mobility on the maxillary left second molar.

guidelines suggest that periodontal health should be achieved in the least invasive and most cost-effective manner possible.[9] In this regard, the appropriate nonsurgical treatment of periodontitis must maximize the inherent healing potential of the periodontal wound, minimizing iatrogenic trauma on dental and soft tissue—and consequently, intra- and posttreatment morbidity.[10]

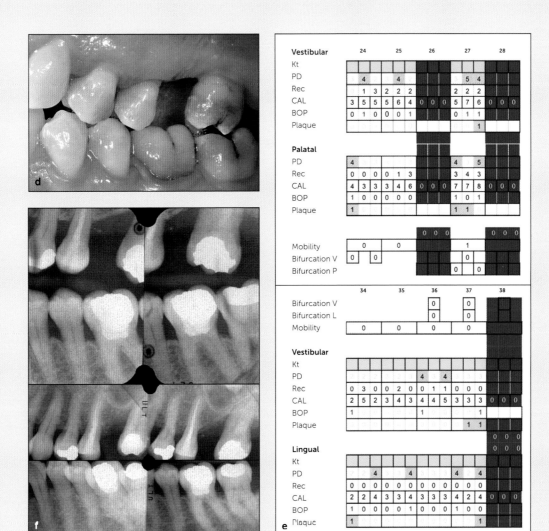

Fig 3-2 (cont) *(d to f)* Clinical and radiographic results 3 years following the completion of nonsurgical therapy. Note the reduction in PD, disappearance of BOP, recovery of the mobility the maxillary second molar, and remineralization of the intrabony component of the defect on the mesial aspect of the maxillary second molar. Kt, keratinized tissue; Rec, recession; CAL, clinical attachment level; V, vestibular; P, palatal; L, lingual.

Nonsurgical periodontal therapy in patients affected by periodontitis has the three following aims:

1. Remove hard and soft deposits to provide a biologically compatible root surface (Fig 3-2)
2. Control microbial infection
3. Reestablish periodontal health[11] (Fig 3-3)

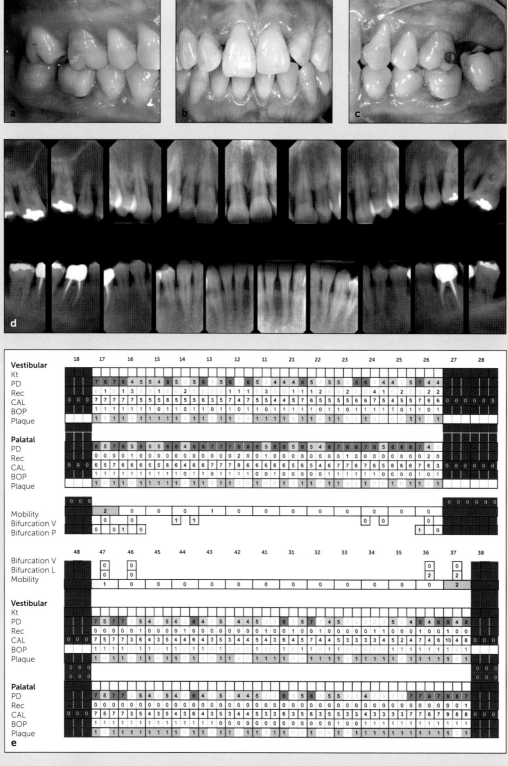

Fig 3-3 A 30-year-old woman with Stage III, Grade C periodontitis. Her medical condition was not contributory. She was a nonsmoker and has a family history of periodontitis. *(a to e)* Clinical photographs, radiographs, and chart at baseline. Note the amount of microbial deposits inconsistent with the severity of periodontal tissue destruction. →

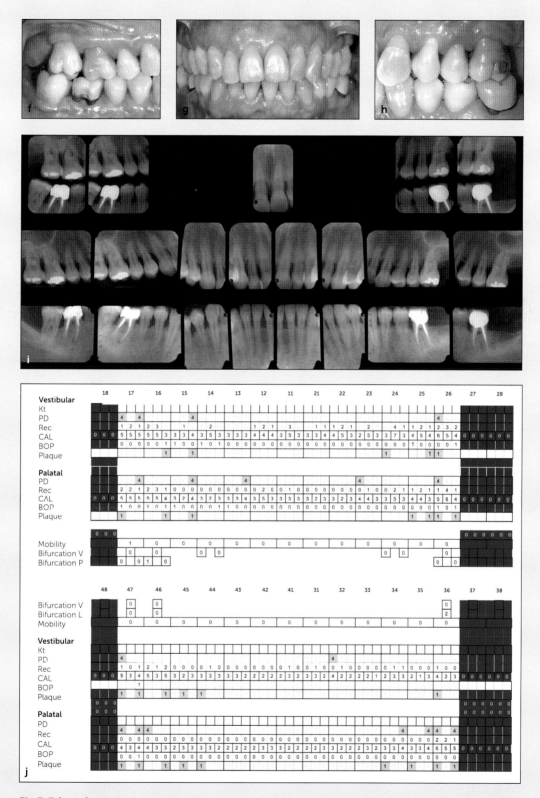

Fig 3-3 (cont) *(f to j)* Clinical photographs, radiographs, and chart at 12-month follow-up. The patient underwent nonsurgical periodontal therapy and then received regular supportive care at 4-month intervals. The recall frequency was based on her susceptibility to periodontitis. During active treatment, pathologically migrated teeth in the second sextant were orthodontically repositioned, and the mandibular left second molar was the only one extracted for periodontal reasons (advanced attachment loss, furcation involvement, Class II mobility) and occlusal reasons (extrusion, interference during eccentric movements, absence of the antagonist). PDs remained at 4 mm on teeth 17, 26, 36, 32, and 47.

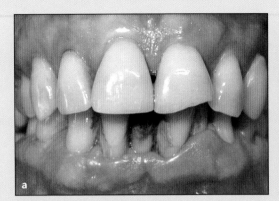
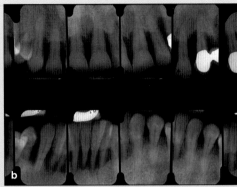

Fig 3-4 *(a and b)* Maxillary and mandibular anterior sextants in a patient with Stage IV, Grade C periodontitis. This patient is also a heavy smoker. Note the thickened fibrotic consistency of the marginal periodontium and tooth staining. Clinical and radiographic examination revealed PD up to 9 mm, advanced bone loss, and reduced gingival bleeding. Clinical signs of poor inflammatory response to local irritants could be attributable to the masking effect of smoking on gingival inflammatory symptoms, providing smokers with a false sense of healthy gingiva. Modification of risk factors is critical to the control of periodontal disease.

During this treatment phase, clinicians should try to change modifiable risk factors, such as smoking habits and poor glycemic control of diabetes mellitus[12] (Fig 3-4). Factors that cannot be modified, including a family history of periodontal diseases or immune diseases, have to be factored into the expected outcomes. The clinician sets the definitive treatment plan based on a comprehensive diagnosis and evaluation of individual response to nonsurgical therapy. Additional corrective surgery of residual pockets or defects may be considered as part of the treatment plan.

Relevance of patient-based plaque control for the regenerative outcome

The success of any periodontal treatment, including regenerative procedures, is dependent on the patient's compliance in self-performed plaque control. A team approach to periodontal treatment can be very successful. The dental hygienist should not only demonstrate professional competence in oral health care but also have a proactive approach in motivating patients. It is important to establish mutual cooperation between the operator and the patient. Individualized oral hygiene instructions should be given to all patients undergoing periodontal therapy and reinforced at each treatment session.[6] Patients are more motivated to accept treatment recommendations when they are given the opportunity to directly perceive the amount and location of plaque deposits in their dentition.[12] One suggestion is first to show the brushing methods in the patient's mouth as professionally performed by the dental hygienist. Then, the patient should be asked to perform the oral hygiene procedures under professional supervision (Fig 3-5).

Many different tooth brushing methods have been suggested, but none has been shown superior to another. The modified Bass technique may be indicated for patients unwilling to use an electric toothbrush.[13] Electric toothbrushes are recommended because they remove more plaque than manual toothbrushes.[14,15] Although there is an additional 11% reduction of plaque and an additional

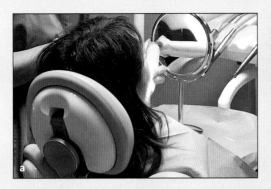
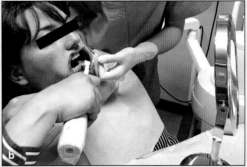

Fig 3-5 *(a and b)* Patients need be aware of their role in dental care. Dental hygienists should reinforce motivation and oral hygiene instruction at each treatment session. Patients should try to perform brushing and flossing under supervision of the dental hygienist. The daily use of a magnifying mirror may assist them in home plaque removal.

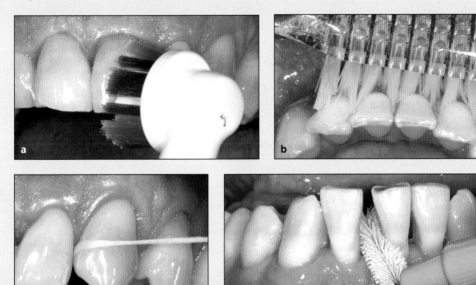

Fig 3-6 *(a to d)* Patients benefit most from individualized instruction in using the toothbrush and interdental devices most suitable for their anatomical conditions.

6% reduction of gingival inflammation at 1 to 3 months following the use of a powered toothbrush, the long-term clinical benefits are still under investigation.[16] Recent data showed comparable effects on gingival recessions following 3-year use of manual versus electric toothbrushes.[17]

Tooth brushing must be coupled with interdental cleaning to effectively remove bacterial biofilm and control gingival inflammation. According to the available evidence, the interdental brush is the most effective device for interproximal cleaning in patients with periodontitis. Flossing is recommended only at periodontally healthy sites where the interdental papilla completely fills the interdental space as well as in all conditions where the interdental brushes do not pass through the interproximal area without causing tissue trauma[18] (Fig 3-6).

The relevance of home-based oral hygiene performance in optimizing the regenerative end points should be carefully shared with the patient because the level of self-performed

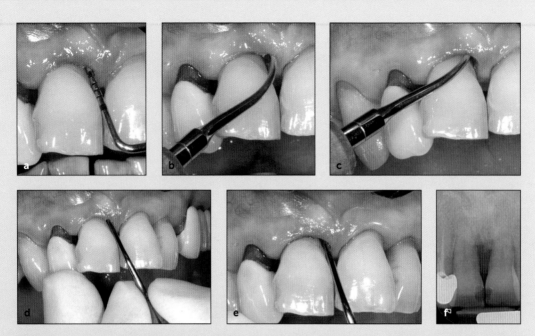

Fig 3-7 The subgingival instrumentation of a periodontal pocket must be always preceded and guided by an accurate diagnosis based on clinical and radiographic data. *(a to e)* These photographs show a maxillary central incisor with a PD of 10 mm on the mesial aspect. The ultrasonic insert and the curette are inserted into the pocket and moved along the root surface from the base of the pocket in a coronal direction to effectively remove soft and hard deposits. *(f)* Preoperative radiograph.

plaque control has shown a robust dose-dependent effect on regenerative procedures. Better clinical attachment level (CAL) gains were reported in patients with optimal levels of supragingival plaque control compared with patients with less ideal oral hygiene.[19]

Methods for successful professional mechanical plaque removal

The supragingival and subgingival dental biofilm and calculus must be mechanically removed to reestablish periodontally healthy conditions. Although epithelial attachment on subgingival calculus has been described in the literature,[20] removal of all subgingival calculus and leaving a smooth root surface are still the clinical end points for professional mechanical plaque removal (PMPR).[21] The current general consensus is that aggressive root surface removal is not needed to achieve a good therapeutic outcome because endotoxins adhere loosely to the root surfaces.[21–23] However, it is very difficult to retain cementum when removing calculus deposits that adhere strictly to the root surface.

The instrumentation must be always guided by the use of a periodontal probe (Fig 3-7). Periodontal probing should always precede and follow the use of hand or ultrasonic devices. It permits clinicians to locate subgingival calculus, measure periodontal pockets, identify tooth anomalies, measure and locate furcation involvement, and check the completeness of the treatment. The use of the periodontal probe should be complemented by a fine-diameter explorer that allows for increased tactile sensitivity in detection of root surface irregularities.

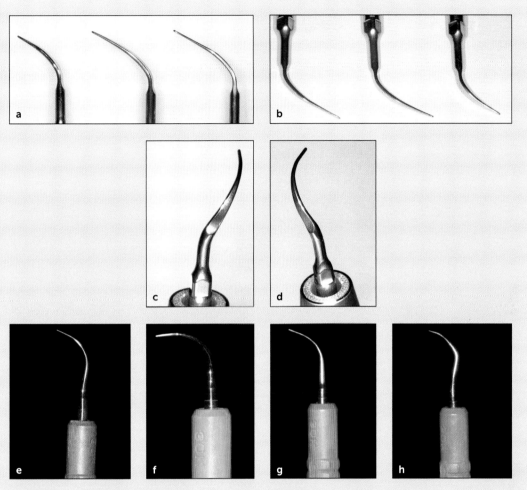

Fig 3-8 Inserts with different curvature and length for piezoelectric and magnetostrictive ultrasonic devices. Ultrasonic scalers operate at a frequency of 18,000 to 45,000 Hz. They have the advantage of the cavitation effect, which occurs when bubbles form in the water and are used as coolant. When these bubbles collapse, they disrupt the cell wall of bacteria. They provide an easier access to the interdental and subgingival area than manual instruments. Wear of the tip affects the working performance of the ultrasonic instrument and therefore should be checked regularly. *(a to d)* Piezoelectric scalers. The strokes occur in a linear pattern via a crystal activated by the ceramic handpiece. Only the lateral sides are effective in removing debris. The most effective instrumentation is performed with the extremity of the tip (ie, the last 2 mm). *(e to h)* Magnetostrictive scalers. The energy is converted in elliptical vibrations of the tip due to a magnetic field in the handpiece that causes the insert to expand and to contract. All surfaces are active in removing debris. Patients are more comfortable due to the mild vibrations.

Manual versus sonic or ultrasonic instruments

The current evidence indicates that none of the available instrumentation techniques are able to completely eliminate subgingival bacteria and calculus. The method to perform PMPR seems to have a limited effect because both ultrasonic or sonic devices and manual instrumentation have been shown to achieve similar clinical and microbiologic results[24,25] (Fig 3-8). The use of manual instruments is considered to be more technically demanding and time-consuming than the use of sonic or ultrasonic devices, but it allows a better tactile sensation and control over the mechanical instrument.[26]

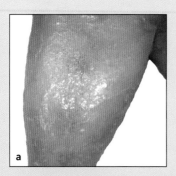
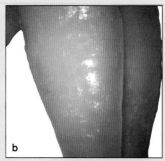

Fig 3-9 Images comparing surface roughness of periodontally diseased molars scaled with powered or hand instrumentation (original magnification ×25). *(a)* Ultrasonic scaler. *(b)* Gracey curette.

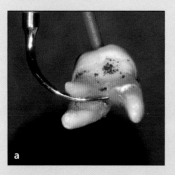
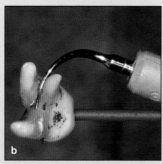
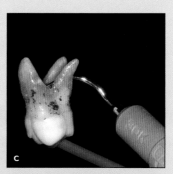

Fig 3-10 *(a to c)* Ultrasonic devices have better access to the interradicular area because they are usually narrower than the furcation entrance. The average width of a furcation is usually less than that of the average hand instrument. The Gracey micro-mini curettes have a thinner and shorter blade for better access into furcation entrances. Curved ultrasonic tips designed for multirooted teeth are available.

Sonic and ultrasonic instruments remove less root structure and cause less soft tissue trauma than mechanical instruments,[24,27] but they seem to create a rougher root surface[28,29] (Fig 3-9). In addition, they produce contaminated aerosols, and some patients may find the vibrations and water spray uncomfortable. On the other hand, the ultrasonic instrumentation has been proven more effective in treating areas with limited access, such as in grade II and III furcation defects[30] (Fig 3-10). Thin ultrasonic inserts have smaller working tips than the smallest curettes, making them a superior choice for calculus removal in moderate to advanced furcation lesions. In the authors' practice, nonsurgical treatment is usually performed with a combination of ultrasonic devices followed by finishing instrumentation with curettes to take advantage of the benefits of both modalities of root instrumentation.[25,31]

Instrument design

The introduction of mini curettes and modified ultrasonic scaler tips (eg, thin, tiny, and periodontal probe–type) has made it easier to reach deeper into the periodontal defects as well as to reduce trauma on dental and soft tissue[24,32] (Fig 3-11). It is fundamental to preserve the architecture of soft tissues during PMPR to minimize the posttreatment recession, thus optimizing the CAL gain and preserving the preexisting esthetics.

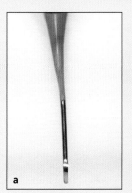 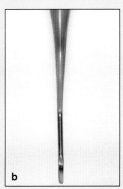 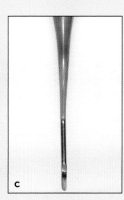 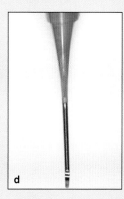

Fig 3-11 Comparison among standard *(a)*, after-five *(b)*, mini *(c)*, and micro-mini *(d)* area-specific Gracey curettes. Gracey curettes with extended shanks and mini or micro-mini blades have been designed to improve the efficacy of subgingival instrumentation. The shorter blade allows easier insertion in deep, tight, and narrow pockets; developmental grooves; furcations; and deep lingual/palatal pockets. They can be used with vertical strokes with reduced tissue distension and without soft tissue trauma.

Local adjunctive treatments

The added benefit from the application of lasers, photodynamic therapy, air polishing, and antimicrobials to treat periodontal pockets remains controversial. Their use seems to only marginally enhance the clinician's ability to effectively remove microbial deposits from the root surfaces and improve clinical outcomes.[33] Adjuncts to subgingival instrumentation provided an additional 0.3-mm increase in CAL gain over 6 to 12 months compared with subgingival instrumentation alone.[34]

Lasers. Laser therapy is generally reported to have bactericidal, ablative, and detoxification effects.[35] The Nd:YAG and diode lasers have limited use in root detoxification or calculus removal because their targets are primarily the soft tissues. Diode laser application can result in soft tissue penetration ranging from about 0.5 to 3 mm and complete removal of pocket epithelium.[36] Thus, it is used for inactivation of bacteria and removal of inflamed soft tissue from periodontal pockets as well for achieving hemostasis in acutely inflamed tissue.[37] Because of less effective removal of deposits as well as the potential thermal damage on the root surface that Nd:YAG and diode lasers might produce, they cannot be used as a replacement for mechanical instruments in root debridement procedures.[38]

The most promising laser for debridement seems to be the Er:YAG laser, which is capable of effectively removing calculus. The absorption of its energy by water and inorganic components favors the detachment of hard deposits from the root surface.[35] It exerts a bactericidal effect against periodontal pathogens[39] and has the potential to remove bacterial endotoxins from diseased surfaces without major injury to tooth substance.[40] It is also possible to gain easy access to complicated anatomical sites because of its light beam radiation.[41] However, there is lack of evidence to support the use of laser as an adjuvant to PMPR or alternative method for nonsurgical treatment of periodontal pockets.[42–44]

Photodynamic therapy. Photodynamic therapy (PDT) is based on the principle that a photosensitizer agent binds to the target cells and is activated through light of a certain wavelength to

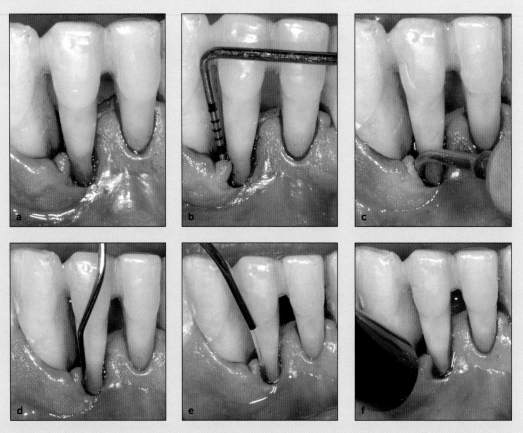

Fig 3-12 Use of laser and PDT in a periodontal pocket on the distal aspect of the mandibular lateral incisor. *(a)* Clinical appearance. *(b)* Preoperative CAL. *(c)* Use of ultrasonic device for subgingival instrumentation. *(d)* Insertion of an explorer to check the smoothness and cleanliness of the root surface. *(e)* Insertion and activation of the diode laser tip. (Operator and patient must wear protective eyeglasses.) *(f)* Application of a cycle of PDT. The adjunctive use of laser and/or PDT does not provide any relevant additional positive effect over routine scaling and root planing (SRP).

generate highly reactive and cytotoxic singlet oxygen, resulting in bacterial cell death.[45] PDT does not remove bacterial biofilm and calculus, and it may not substantially suppress pathogenic bacteria in periodontal pockets.[46] Available evidence shows that PDT does not provide an additional positive effect in the management of periodontitis over routine mechanical treatment[47] (Fig 3-12).

Air polishing. The application of air polishing has been also suggested as an adjunctive treatment approach for supragingival and subgingival instrumentation. Sodium bicarbonate air polishing devices have been proven efficient in supragingival polishing and stain removal, but they are not suitable for subgingival use because of significant root substance removal and damage during application.[48,49] Low-abrasive amino acid glycine powder air polishing has been introduced to overcome this limitation. It is effective in removing the subgingival biofilm by minimizing trauma to hard and soft tissue, but it does not remove mineralized bacterial deposits.[50] Erythritol, a naturally derived sugar alcohol, has recently been introduced in a low-abrasiveness powder with a smaller particle size than glycine. Air polishing with erythritol failed to remove both supra- and subgingival hard calculus deposits, and its effectiveness was comparable with glycine air polishing for removal of soft deposits.[51]

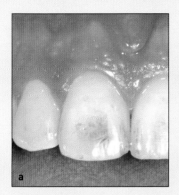 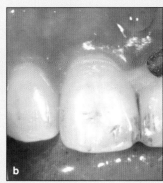 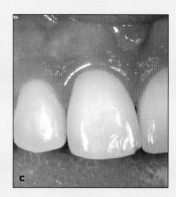

Fig 3-13 Handheld polishing device. The interaction of solid particles with the surface to be treated is the basic process by which abrasive water jets work. The ability of the jet of air, powder, and water to remove stains and bacterial biofilm is influenced to a large degree by the properties of the particles applied, such as shape, geometric form, and hardness. *(a)* Clinical situation before treatment. *(b)* Treatment. *(c)* Immediately after treatment.

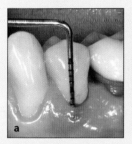 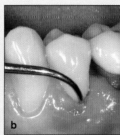 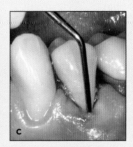 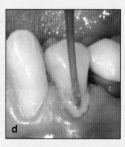

Fig 3-14 Application of doxycycline gel. *(a)* PD of 7 mm in conjunction with BOP on the buccal aspect of the mandibular second premolar with periodontal abscess. *(b)* Use of ultrasonic scaling to remove calculus. *(c)* Insertion of an explorer to check the smoothness of the root surface. *(d)* Application of the antimicrobial agent into the site.

Clinicians are cautioned not to direct the air spray toward the soft tissue wall of the pocket, because this can cause subcutaneous facial emphysema.[52] Moreover, the use of air polishing may be contraindicated close to extraction sites and in cases with extensive loss of bony support and very deep periodontal pockets.[51] Therefore, for calculus removal and initial nonsurgical periodontal therapy, manual and power-driven devices are still the instruments of choice[53,54] (Fig 3-13). In periodontal maintenance therapy, air polishing showed clinical outcomes comparable with ultrasonic and manual debridement.[51] Previous studies have demonstrated that only 4.7% of the subgingival root surfaces were covered with calculus after 3 months of recolonization in instrumented teeth.[55]

Antimicrobials. Local application of antimicrobials (including antibiotics and antiseptics), allowing the minimum inhibitory concentration of the drug to be available for a prolonged period of time, has been advocated for patients with localized lesions or nonresponding and recurrent sites.[56] Local antibiotics include a 10% doxycycline gel in a bioabsorbable mixture that maintains its activity for 21 days, a 14% doxycycline gel that releases the drug for up to 12 days (Fig 3-14), and a powder containing 1 mg of minocycline spheres that maintains its activity over a period of 14 days. Compared with systemic antibiotic therapy,

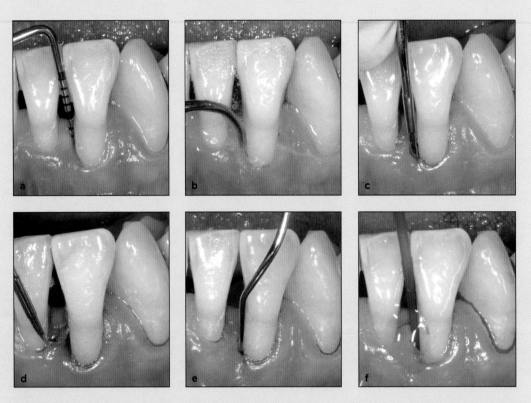

Fig 3-15 Subgingival irrigation with 1% chlorhexidine gel after the completion of SRP with hand and ultrasonic devices. *(a)* Deep periodontal pocket on the mesial aspect of the mandibular lateral incisor. *(b)* Subgingival instrumentation with ultrasonic device. *(c and d)* Subgingival instrumentation with Gracey curettes. *(e)* Use of the explorer to check the completeness of the instrumentation. *(f)* Irrigation of the periodontal pocket with 1% chlorhexidine gel.

local antimicrobials cause fewer adverse effects, have lower risk of developing bacterial resistance, and have better patient compliance. However, the adjunctive application of locally delivered antibiotics seems to achieve only minor benefits: an additional 0.4 to 0.6 mm of probing depth (PD) reduction[57,58] and an additional CAL gain of up to 0.3 mm can be expected.[59,60] Two systematic reviews suggested that local antimicrobials combined with scaling and root planning (SRP) improve PD and CAL at sites with baseline PD of ≥ 5 mm in smokers[61] and in diabetic patients affected by periodontitis.[62] However, heterogeneity among studies prevents a clear assessment of the usefulness of topical antimicrobials, and the clinical relevance of the observed clinical improvements is questionable.

It is also possible to use chlorhexidine gluconate, an antiseptic that binds reversibly to oral and tooth surfaces with low release, which allows for a sustained antimicrobial effect (for up to 12 hours). When used as an adjunct to nonsurgical treatment, chlorhexidine rinse resulted in additional reduction of supragingival plaque and delayed bacterial recolonization compared with periodontal instrumentation alone.[63] In contrast, subgingival chlorhexidine irrigation would seem not to significantly improve the results of the nonsurgical periodontal treatment because it might not be retained long enough in the periodontal pocket for its pharmacologic

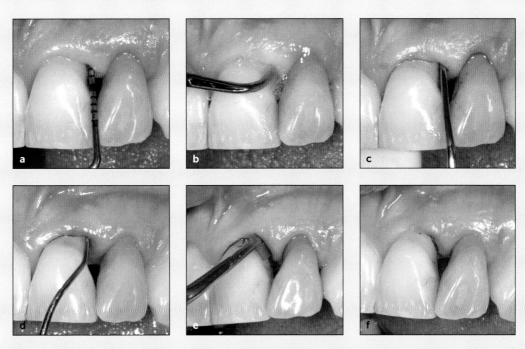

Fig 3-16 Insertion of a chlorhexidine chip into a deep periodontal pocket. *(a)* PD of 8 mm on the distal aspect of a maxillary central incisor. *(b)* Subgingival instrumentation with ultrasonic device. *(c)* Subgingival instrumentation with a 5/6 Gracey mini five curette. *(d)* Use of an explorer to check the completeness of the subgingival PMPR. The side of the curved tip of the explorer was adapted to the contour of the tooth surface and moved repeatedly in apicocoronal vertical and oblique strokes to detect subgingival dental calculus and root irregularities. The flexible and fine-pointed tip enhances the accuracy in detecting subgingival hard deposits compared with the periodontal probe. *(e)* Insertion of a chlorhexidine chip. The chip releases chlorhexidine in a biphasic manner, initially releasing approximately 40% of the chlorhexidine within the first 24 hours and then releasing the remaining chlorhexidine for 7 to 10 days due to the enzymatic degradation of the carrier. *(f)* Clinical photograph at the completion of the nonsurgical treatment.

effect to occur.[33,64] Chlorhexidine is also available in gels with concentrations higher than in solution to deliver in periodontal pockets. However, there was no statistical or clinical advantage for their use[58,65] (Fig 3-15). In spite of the viscosity of the gel, it was found that 20 mL/h flow of gingival fluid leads to 1-minute half-life of the medication in periodontal pockets.[66]

To overcome this limit, a 2.5-mg chlorhexidine biodegradable chip (PerioChip) has been introduced that releases the drug for up to 7 to 10 days (Fig 3-16). However, the magnitude of additional clinical benefit is modest compared with conventional debridement alone.[59,60] A recent systematic review reported an added benefit of PerioChip of 0.4 mm in CAL over subgingival instrumentation alone.[33] Thus, the clinician should take into account the previously described limitations and the cost-efficacy ratio when making a clinical decision.[67]

Clinical outcomes of nonsurgical therapy

The efficacy of PMPR combined with proper self-performed plaque control in treating periodontitis has been widely demonstrated in systematic reviews.[33,68] It results in reduction

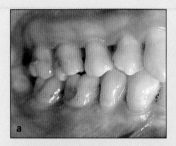
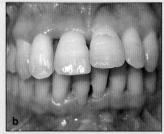
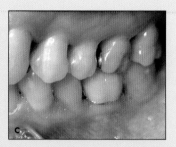
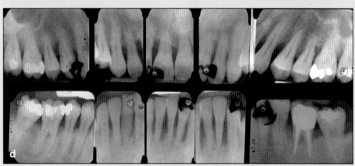
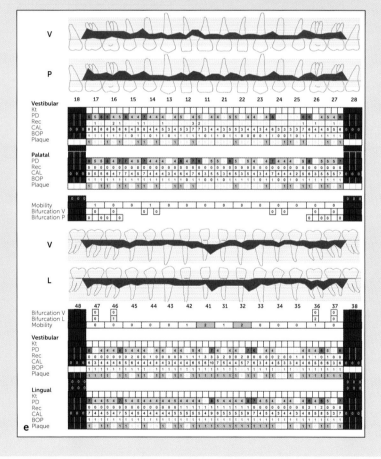

Fig 3-17 This young woman was healthy with a family history of periodontitis. She presented with Stage IV, Grade C periodontitis with tooth mobility in the second and fifth sextants and pathologic migration of the maxillary anterior teeth. *(a to e)* In 2002, she underwent a single-stage full-mouth disinfection according to the protocol by Quirynen et al[70] modified by Bollen et al[71] in association with systemic antibiotic administration (amoxicillin and metronidazole).[72,73] Occlusal adjustment was performed at each recall visit.

of inflammation, as indicated by the disappearance or reduction of bleeding on probing (BOP), decreased PD, and CAL gain. Another parameter to be considered is the reduction of tooth mobility.[12] Nonsurgical periodontal therapy may also contribute to spontaneous correction of pathologic tooth migration and closure of diastema[69] (Fig 3-17).[70–73]

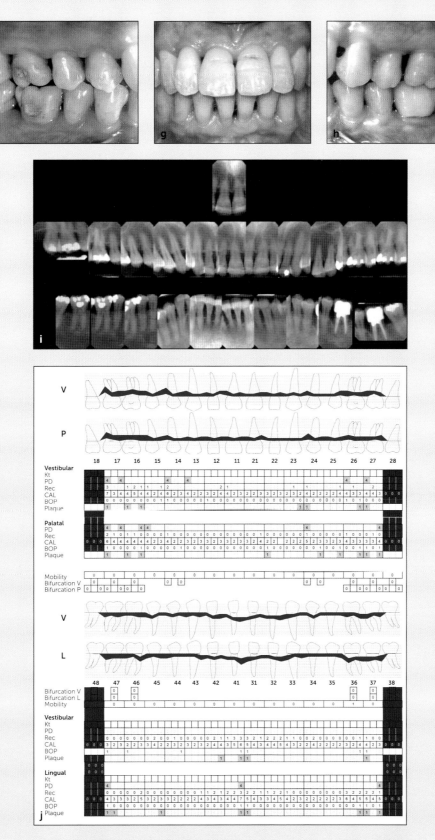

Fig 3-17 (cont) *(f to j)* Spontaneous repositioning of maxillary anterior teeth was obtained progressively during the first 2 years following nonsurgical therapy. Note also the radiographic remineralization of the lamina dura. ⟶

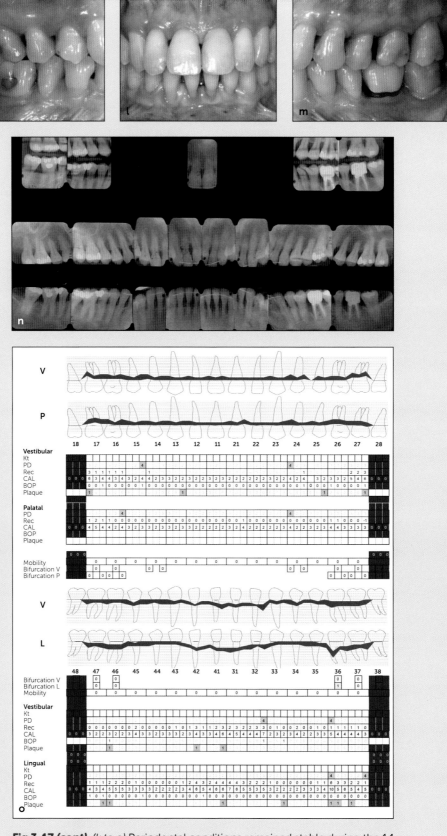

Fig 3-17 (cont) *(k to o)* Periodontal conditions remained stable during the 14 years of supportive periodontal therapy.

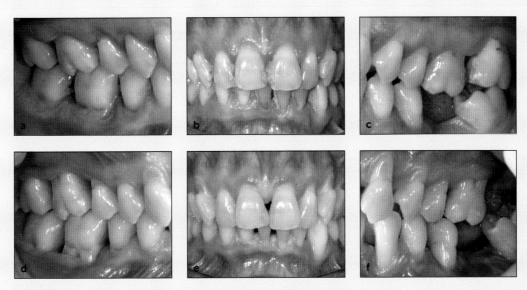

Fig 3-18 *(a to c)* Note the poor oral hygiene with plaque and calculus deposits in the interdental area of the majority of teeth prior to nonsurgical therapy. *(d to f)* Following treatment, the shrinkage of gingival tissue is particularly evident at the premolar and molar sites. The amount of recession is mainly related to the initial severity of PD and gingival phenotype.

Posttreatment PD reduction can in be attributed part to both the shrinkage of the soft tissues, leading to a recession of the gingival margin, and decreased probe penetration into the pocket. This is caused by the resolution of the inflammatory process as well as the regained density of connective fibers still inserted into the root cementum at the most apical part of the defect.[74] Soft tissue recession is a common observation at most sites following nonsurgical instrumentation, particularly when the tissues are highly inflamed and edematous and/or in the presence of a thin gingival phenotype (Fig 3-18). Deeper pockets and thinner gingival phenotypes exhibit greater posttreatment recession.

The outcome of PMPR is strictly dependent on the initial PD.[33,68,75] Subgingival instrumentation should be avoided at sites with PD ≤ 3 mm to prevent attachment loss due to tissue trauma.[76] In this context, the term *critical probing depth* defines the minimal PD suitable for subgingival PMPR.[76] At moderate sites (ie, PD of 4 to 6 mm), clinicians should expect a mean PD reduction of about 1 mm and a CAL gain of approximately 0.5 mm.[33,68,75] At deeper pockets (ie, PD ≥ 7 mm), the PD reduction averages approximately 2 mm, and CAL gain is approximately 1 mm.[33,68,75] PD reduction is expected to be 0.5 mm less in molar sites with grade II or III furcation involvement.[77]

The clinical end point of treatment success in the reevaluation following nonsurgical therapy should be stability—or at least remission or control—of the periodontal disease.[78] Ideally, restoration of periodontal stability should be a major treatment goal and can be attained through a strict control of inflammation and infection as well as of any local and systemic modifying factors, resulting in complete resolution of inflammation or minimal BOP and normal gingival sulcus depth.[78] While periodontal stability should be a clear treatment target, an acceptable alternative therapeutic goal may be low disease activity. This can be demonstrated by significant reduction in BOP even without normal gingival sulcus

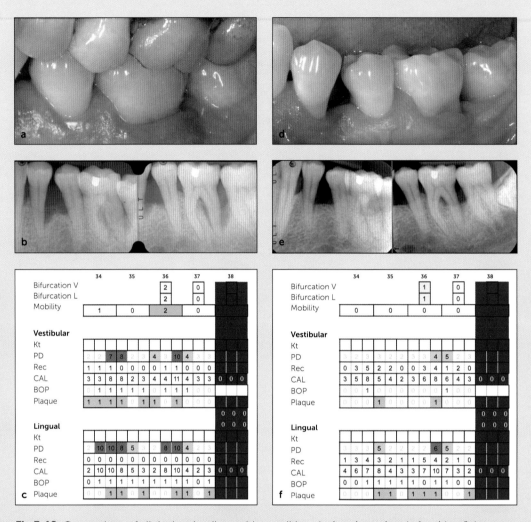

Fig 3-19 Comparison of clinical and radiographic conditions before *(a to c)* and after *(d to f)* the completion of nonsurgical therapy in the fourth sextant. Note the spontaneous remineralization of the intrabony defects on both premolars and first molar after 2 years. As reported in the periodontal chart, the treatment has been effective in reducing PD, improving furcation involvements, and achieving complete recovery of dental stability. Nonetheless, some sites exhibit persisting BOP.

depth, particularly in patients with long-standing disease and/or uncontrolled contributing factors, such as smoking and diabetes mellitus[78] (Fig 3-19). Absence of BOP has been shown to be an excellent indicator of periodontal stability,[79] and pocket closure (ie, a conversion of a pocket into a nonbleeding site with PD of ≤ 4 mm) is associated with lower risk of disease progression and tooth loss.[80,81]

In contrast, posttreatment residual pockets exhibiting BOP and a PD of 5 or 6 mm are associated with a lower clinical stability with an odds ratio for disease progression of 7.7 and 11.0, respectively, compared with a site with PD of ≤ 3 mm.[80] The odds ratio increases to 64.2 for residual PD ≥ 7 mm.[80] Sites demonstrating persisting BOP exhibit about 40% to 75% more attachment loss per year than healthy and slightly inflamed sites[82]; for teeth consistently surrounded by inflamed gingiva, the risk of tooth loss is 46 times higher.[83]

Fig 3-20 *(a)* Anatomical aberration on the furcation entrance of a mandibular first molar. *(b)* Root groove on a mandibular second premolar. Abnormal anatomical characteristics may increase dental biofilm accumulation, may be an obstacle to appropriate root instrumentation, and may contribute to local deepening of periodontal pockets. Many failures in periodontal treatment are related to inadequate evaluation of teeth with distinct anatomical characteristics and incorrect diagnosis.

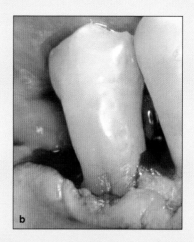

Fig 3-21 Residual calculus on the root surface of the maxillary *(a)* and mandibular *(b)* second molars. Complete calculus removal is rarely achieved with SRP. Periodontal pockets with 4 to 6 mm PD still have 15% to 40% of the root surface covered by deposits, and those deeper than 6 mm have 19% to 66% covered following subgingival instrumentation.

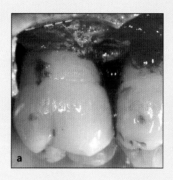 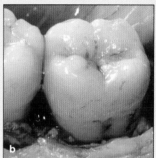

Limitations of subgingival PMPR

Limitations of subgingival PMPR are well documented. Its efficacy seems to be related to operator skill; defect morphology; complex tooth anatomy, such as root invagination or grooves, enamel pearls, or projections; and width of the interdental space[84] (Fig 3-20). On average, about 35% of initially pathologic pockets may not reach the end point of treatment success.[85]

Residual calculus has been found in 23% of 5- to 6-mm pockets and in 35% of pockets deeper than 6 mm. Clinical and radiographic improvement is generally less pronounced at molar and furcation sites, possibly in part because 30% of multirooted teeth versus 10% of single-rooted teeth still present residual calculus following PMPR[86–88] (Fig 3-21).

Clinical outcomes are also impaired by patient-related factors such as poor self-performed plaque control, smoking habits, and uncontrolled diabetes mellitus[84] (Fig 3-22). Smoking habits influence treatment response at deep pocket sites. Smokers have a probability of pocket closure of 36% versus 67% in nonsmokers when considering pockets with an initial PD of 7 mm.[89] Obese patients may also experience a worse healing response after nonsurgical treatment in moderate to deep pockets.[90]

Interestingly, reinstrumentation of sites that responded poorly to the nonsurgical treatment is successful in only 11% to 16% of the pockets,[88] and the probability of pocket closure in pockets > 6 mm is 12%.[89] Thus, in persistently deep residual pockets, a surgical correction may be recommended.

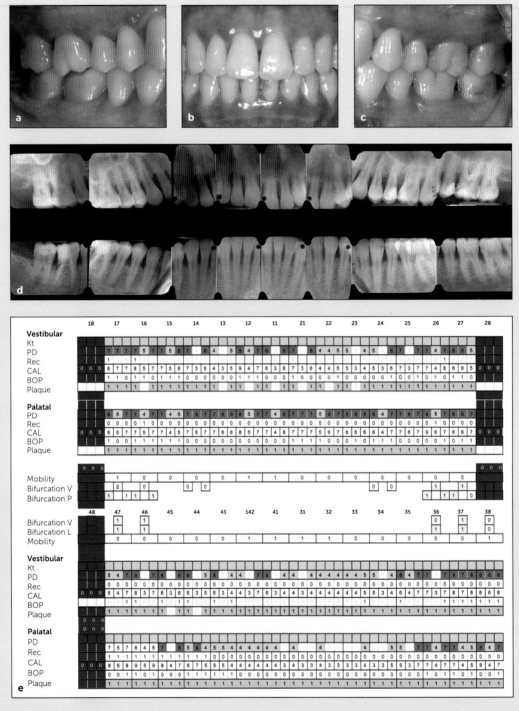

Fig 3-22 Clinical and radiographic presentation of a 29-year-old woman with type 1 diabetes. The patient was diagnosed with diabetes mellitus at the age of 17 years, has poor glycemic control, and smokes more than 20 cigarettes per day. *(a to e)* Periodontal examination at baseline revealed generalized severe periodontitis with PDs ranging between 4 and 9 mm on most teeth and multiple sites with bacterial plaque and clinical signs of inflammation. During the nonsurgical periodontal therapy, the patient stopped smoking, and in spite of the improvement in plaque control (full-mouth plaque score, FMPS) and the decrease in the percentage of sites with BOP (full-mouth bleeding score, FMBS) compared with the corresponding baseline values, periodontal conditions deteriorated significantly. The number of deep pocket sites remained high, and some interradicular lesions appeared on the maxillary molars.

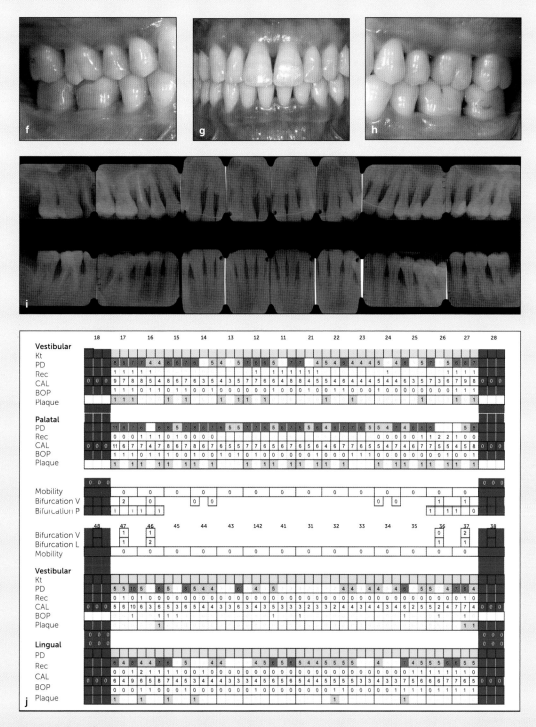

Fig 3-22 (cont) *(f to j)* The response to therapy after 3 years may be impaired by her poor glycemic control (HbA1c unstable and often more than 7%).

Patient reevaluation after nonsurgical therapy

In general, clinicians should assess post-PMPR healing 6 to 8 weeks after treatment.[91] The reestablishment of junctional epithelium is complete within 2 weeks, while the repair of connective tissue occurs within 4 to 8 weeks.[91] However, tissue maturation may continue for an additional 9 to 12 months or longer. Badersten et al[92] reported that the deeper the site, the longer it took to achieve maximal healing. According to available evidence, reevaluation of results should be carried out at least 6 months after the completion of nonsurgical treatment before considering the indication for periodontal regenerative therapy.[93]

MINIMALLY INVASIVE NONSURGICAL THERAPY FOR INTRAOSSEOUS DEFECTS

Rationale of a nonsurgical approach to intraosseous defects

In recent years, a growing interest for more patient-oriented interventions has moved dentistry toward less invasive procedures to reduce operative trauma while still achieving a satisfactory therapeutic result. A special emphasis has been focused on the design and performance of surgical procedures for periodontal regeneration of intrabony defects. Specific surgical approaches have been proposed with the aim to produce minimal wounds, minimal flap reflection, and gentle handling of the soft and hard tissues (see chapter 4).

Due to increased availability of magnification systems, dental endoscopes, and microsurgical instruments, this minimally invasive approach has led to the development of less invasive instrumentation principles even in nonsurgical periodontal therapy.[10,94] A recent randomized controlled study stressed the aspects of the retention of the preoperative gingival architecture and of gentle handling of periodontal tissue according to a minimally invasive nonsurgical protocol.[95,96] A negligible morbidity and similar PD reduction and CAL gain were reported when comparing the clinical performance of minimally invasive surgical and minimally invasive nonsurgical therapy (MINST) in the treatment of deep intraosseous defects.

Treatment protocol for intraosseous defects

Among nonsurgical treatment options, MINST has been recently introduced as a concept aiming to obtain extensive subgingival debridement with minimal soft tissue trauma and minimal patient morbidity during the closed instrumentation of intraosseous defects.[95–97] When performing the MINST protocol, the recommendations listed in Box 3-1 should be followed.[96–98]

To ensure extensive subgingival debridement, the selected instrumentation must be easy to insert in the periodontal pocket and should reach the entire extension of the exposed and contaminated root surface. Thus, an extensive subgingival root debridement, from the gingival margin up to the bottom of the periodontal pocket, may be effectively obtained by using specific instrumentation such as ultrasonic devices with thin and delicate tips that may be eventually complemented by mini curettes (eg, Gracey mini curettes from after five to micro mini five). During periodontal debridement, the aim is to be as conservative as possible—

> **Box 3-1 Recommendations for the MINST protocol**
>
> - Provide a local anesthetic at the defect to be treated.
> - Use magnification systems such as 3.5× loupes[97] or a surgical microscope.[96,99]
> - Select the appropriate instrumentation to minimize the trauma to soft tissues (ie, ultrasonic devices with specific thin and delicate tips complemented by Gracey mini curettes).
> - Debride the root surface to the bottom of the periodontal pocket, avoiding any trauma on hard and soft tissue.
> - Avoid subgingival irrigation.
> - Schedule patient recalls every 2 to 3 months for oral hygiene instructions and supra- and subgingival debridement.

to remove all the mineralized and nonmineralized dental biofilm without intentionally removing cementum and/or dentin from the root surface to obtain a smoother surface. In this context, the use of a magnification system such as loupes or a microscope is mandatory: An enlarged view allows for careful movements that can respect the root surface anatomy.[95]

A second prerequisite of MINST is to produce minimal soft tissue trauma to subsequently minimize posttreatment gingival recession. Limited recession following instrumentation may enhance the CAL gain while reducing the esthetic impact of the treatment. Again, such a minimally invasive approach should be largely based on the ultrasonic instrumentation, eventually complemented by Gracey mini curettes. It is of utmost importance for the manual instrumentation to exclude any direct action on the soft tissue wall of the pocket (ie, gingival curettage). A specific aim of MINST is to stimulate the spontaneous formation of a stable blood clot by allowing the intraosseous defect to naturally fill with blood following debridement.[96] For this reason, the use of subgingival irrigation at the completion of root instrumentation is discouraged.

After MINST, patients are recalled every 2 to 3 months for oral hygiene instructions and supra- and subgingival PMPR.[97,99] At 12 months after the initial instrumentation, the treatment outcome is assessed with clinical and radiographic examination.[96]

Clinical results of MINST

MINST protocol has been shown to result in a substantial treatment response in deep intraosseous defects. After 12 months following treatment, the average PD reduction is 3.1 mm, while the average CAL gain ranged from 2.6 to 3.1 mm.[96,97] These results were paralleled by a slight increase in gingival recession, varying from 0.3 mm[97] to 0.5 mm.[96] A radiographic bone fill of 2.9 mm was also observed in defects with an average intrabony component of 6.7 mm.[96] These clinical and radiographic results were shown to remain stable over a period of 5 years, given that appropriate maintenance care is provided.[99]

MINST appears to lead to enhanced CAL gain when historically compared with SRP procedures in intraosseous defects. Although promising, clinical results following MINST must be interpreted with caution because they are based on intraosseous lesions with an initial moderate PD (mean PD range of 6.4 to 7.8 mm). Moreover, no studies are currently available to determine whether and to what extent MINST shows a clinical superiority to conventional subgingival PMPR in the treatment of deep intraosseous defects.

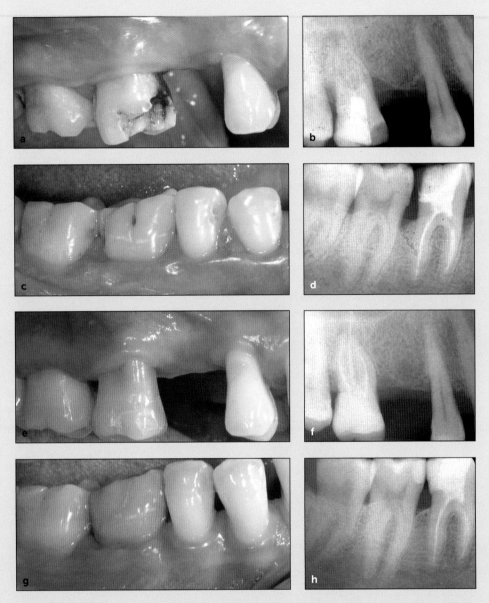

Fig 3-23 Clinical and radiographic appearance of periodontal pockets distal to the maxillary first premolar and mesial to the maxillary first molar and the mandibular first and second molars. *(a to d)* Before the nonsurgical therapy. *(e to h)* Three years after the completion of the nonsurgical therapy. Note the almost complete radiographic closure of the bony defects and the remineralization of the lamina dura. The endodontic treatment of the maxillary first molar could have contributed to the resolution of the previous angular defect, and the restorative treatment had a protective role on the mesial marginal ridge.

Regenerative potential of MINST

The ultimate goal of periodontal treatment has always been regeneration of lost periodontal tissue. Space provision and clot stability during the early healing phase are key elements for successful and predictable regeneration in intrabony defects.[100,101] The blood clot stability prevents the apical migration of the epithelial cells during the first days of healing, and the fibrin clot contains growth factors involved in the periodontal regenerative process.[102,103] Minimally invasive approaches for

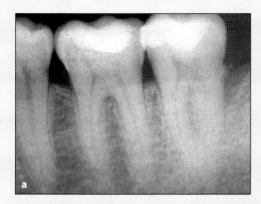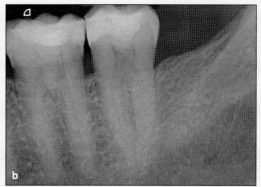

Fig 3-24 Intrabony defect on the distal aspect of a mandibular second molar. *(a)* Baseline. *(b)* Radiographic bone fill at 2-year reevaluation after minimally invasive nonsurgical treatment.

nonsurgical treatment of intraosseous defects might enhance blood clot stability while achieving and maintaining soft tissue architecture (Fig 3-23).

Although radiographically nonsurgical treatment may result in reappearance of the lamina dura and bone remineralization of the intraosseous component[104] (Fig 3-24), experimental studies and human biopsies generally show the formation of a junctional epithelium interposed between the newly formed bone and the root surface.[105,106] Therefore, complete radiographic bone fill does not necessarily reflect periodontal regeneration.

Human biopsies taken at different observation intervals following a single episode of SRP showed that the presence of residual deposits was associated with persistent signs of chronic soft tissue inflammation and no signs of osteoblastic deposition in the alveolar crest.[107] In MINST approaches, the removal of plaque and calculus from intrabony pockets has usually been assisted by the use of magnifying devices, dedicated instruments (eg, micro mirrors and soft tissue retractors), and optimal illumination. Improvement in dental biofilm removal with closed access might create more favorable environmental conditions for periodontal regeneration to occur. Histologic evidence for new bone formation has been reported on extracted teeth 6 months following a single episode of closed SRP assisted by a dental endoscope, associated with absence of signs of chronic inflammation and presence of long junctional epithelium.[108]

THE FLAPLESS PROCEDURE

The flapless procedure (FP) consists of a combination of MINST protocol with the use of enamel matrix derivatives (EMD).[109] The rationale to use EMD with a closed (ie, nonsurgical) procedure is to maximize the natural regenerative potential of the residual intrabony defects by applying a biologic mediator involved in cell differentiation processes in a space filled with a blood clot.[110] Also, the preservation of soft tissue walls while enhancing blood clot stability overcomes a limitation of EMD: Its gel-like consistency may not provide sufficient soft tissue or flap support, potentially limiting the space available for the regeneration process.[111]

EMD may function as potential epithelial-mesenchymal signaling molecules during tooth development.[110] Findings from histologic studies performed in animals and humans have provided

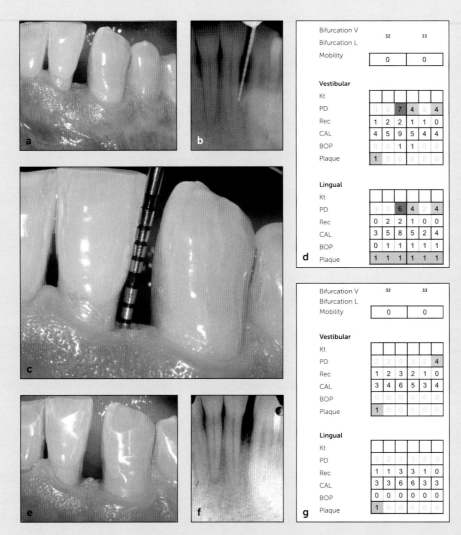

Fig 3-25 Clinical and radiographic aspects of an intrabony defect on the distal aspect of a mandibular lateral incisor before *(a to d)* and 2 years after *(e to g)* FP with EMD. Note the resolution of the intrabony component of the defect.

evidence for periodontal regeneration (ie, formation of cementum, periodontal ligament, and alveolar bone) following EMD treatment.[112] Clinically, local application of EMD in intraosseous periodontal defects has been shown to result in clinical improvements in terms of CAL gain and PD reduction, greater than open flap debridement alone and comparable with other more technically demanding regenerative procedures, such as guided tissue regeneration.[113–115]

A recent randomized clinical trial demonstrated that FPs may be successfully applied in the regenerative treatment of deep intraosseous defects, leading to clinical outcomes comparable with those of minimally invasive surgical approaches. In defects treated with the FP, a mean PD reduction of 3.6 ± 1.0 mm and a CAL gain of 3.2 ± 1.1 mm were observed. In the minimally invasive surgery group, these measurements were 3.7 ± 0.6 mm and 3.6 ± 0.9 mm, respectively (Fig 3-25). In contrast, the radiographic bone fill at 24 months was greater in the surgically treated sites (3.8 ± 1.3 mm versus 2.6 ± 1.6 mm). However, comparable outcomes were obtained with anterior teeth, and comparable patient-oriented outcomes were observed for all teeth. Furthermore, the closed approach may present important advantages in terms of reduction of the operative chair time.[98]

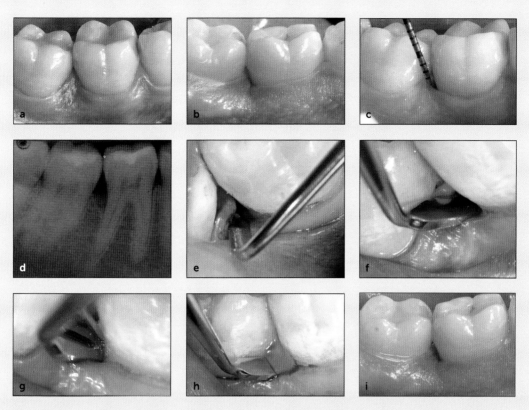

Fig 3-26 Preoperative patient and site preparation. A critical prerequisite to periodontal regeneration is the control of periodontal infection. The patient should present with low levels of plaque and inflammation as the result of successful cause-related therapy (FMPS and FMBS < 10%). The patient should not smoke, and systemic diseases have to be under control. Buccal *(a)* and lingual *(b)* aspects of the mandibular first molar at 6-month reevaluation after conventional nonsurgical therapy. Diagnosis of residual intrabony defect following nonsurgical therapy is based on periodontal probing and radiographs. The radiographic examination must be correlated with clinical findings. The difference in CAL between the interproximal surfaces of the two neighboring teeth represents the intrabony component of the defect. The periapical radiograph provides relevant information about the morphology of the defect. *(c)* The distal surface of the first molar has a CAL of 6 mm, and the mesial surface of the second molar has a CAL of 2 mm; the depth of the intrabony component is 4 mm. *(d)* The radiograph shows a two-walled defect. *(e and f)* The flapless procedure. After local anesthesia, the flapless approach requires a careful removal of residual calculus before the regenerative material is placed. The indirect visualization of the subgingival margin of the root surface is accomplished under an operating microscope at 12.5× magnification with the aid of a gingival retractor and a microsurgical dental mirror. The gingival retractor *(e)* gently displaces the marginal soft tissue enough to allow the insertion of the dental mirror *(f)*, which provides a view of the working field. This allows the clinician to locate and to evaluate the extent and nature of the subgingival deposits. *(g)* Site debridement. The root surface is thoroughly scaled and root planed by the combined action of micro curettes and ultrasonic devices with thin and delicate tips to minimize trauma to the marginal soft tissue. The repeated use of magnifying devices and a tissue retractor facilitates the removal of residual subgingival deposits. *(h)* Application of EMD. Ethylenediaminetetraacetic acid (EDTA) is applied on the instrumented and dried root surfaces for 2 minutes. After that, the defect area is carefully rinsed with saline. Finally, EMD is immediately applied on the dried root surface. *(i)* Soft tissues at the end of the flapless procedure. Caution is taken to preserve the stability of soft tissues with a gentle compression of the gingival margin by means of sterile wetting gauzes until marginal closure of the pocket is attained.

Operative protocol for the FP

The sequences of FP are described step by step in Fig 3-26. A video of the procedures is also available (Video 3-1).

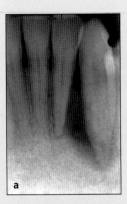 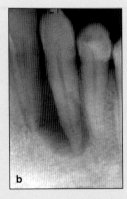 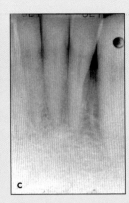 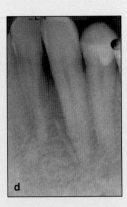

Fig 3-27 *(a and b)* Radiographs at baseline. *(c and d)* Radiographs 3 years after FP. There has been complete resolution of the intrabony component of the defect on the mesial aspect of the canine.

Posttreatment regimen following FP

At completion of FP, the patient is dismissed with the following prescription:

- One 600-mg tablet of ibuprofen immediately after the regenerative procedure and as needed thereafter
- No mechanical plaque control for 2 weeks
- 0.12% chlorhexidine digluconate mouthrinse for 1 minute, three times per day, for the first 4 weeks
- Weekly recall for professional prophylaxis during the first month and thereafter at 3-month intervals

Potential advantages and limitations of FP

Based on the available clinical evidence, FP can be successfully used in the treatment of intraosseous defects (Figs 3-27 to 3-31). The advantage is to optimize the clinical condition of the intrabony pocket while reducing chair time and treatment costs. The preserved soft tissue of the pocket walls may ensure blood clot stability, whereas the application of EMD would enhance the biologic regenerative potential of the periodontal lesion. Although in principle, the technique might favor the wound healing conditions leading to periodontal regeneration, there is currently no evidence that the clinical benefit is histologically associated with new formation of bone, cementum, and periodontal ligament.

FP also presents some limitations. These include the limited visibility and the technical difficulty in managing defects in the posterior area.[98] In this context, the tooth anatomy and the width of the interdental space may be relevant factors affecting the treatment outcome. As previously stated, FP requires the use of a magnifying system or an operating microscope supplied with adequate coaxial illumination of the operative area. This allows for the direct visualization of the root surface and facilitates the identification and removal of subgingival deposits by dedicated mechanical and hand instruments. This implies specific training whose learning curve has yet not been established.

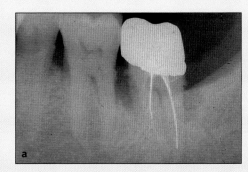
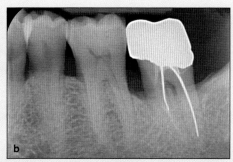

Fig 3-28 *(a)* Radiograph at baseline. *(b)* Radiograph 2 years after FP. In spite of the poor endodontic and restorative treatment, an almost complete bone fill of the intrabony defect was achieved on the mesial aspect of the second molar.

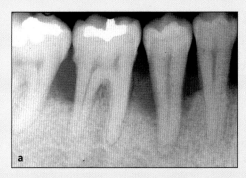
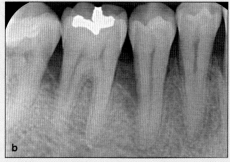

Fig 3-29 Preoperative *(a)* and 1-year follow-up *(b)* radiographic views of the intraosseous defects on the mesial and distal aspects of the second premolar. Note the complete resolution of the defect on the mesial aspect treated with FP.

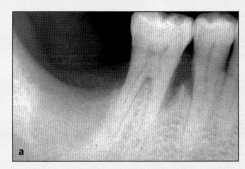
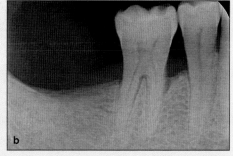

Fig 3-30 *(a)* Baseline radiograph. *(b)* The radiograph 2 years after FP shows the almost complete resolution of the intraosseous defect mesial to the first molar.

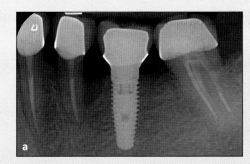
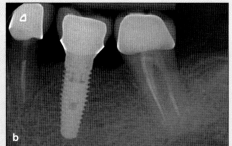

Fig 3-31 *(a)* The baseline radiograph shows the defect on the distal aspect of the second premolar. *(b)* The 2-year follow-up radiograph shows the resolution of the intrabony component of the defect treated with FP (courtesy of Dr Filippo Citterio).

REFERENCES

1. Kornman KS. Mapping the pathogenesis of periodontitis: A new look. J Periodontol 2008;79(8 suppl):1560–1568.

2. Roberts FA, Darveau RP. Microbial protection and virulence in periodontal tissue as a function of polymicrobial communities: Symbiosis and dysbiosis. Periodontol 2000 2015;69:18–27.

3. Bartold PM, Van Dyke TE. Periodontitis: A host-mediated disruption of microbial homeostasis. Unlearning learned concepts. Periodontol 2000 2013;62:203–217.

4. Nunn ME. Understanding the etiology of periodontitis: An overview of periodontal risk factors. Periodontol 2000 2003;32:11–23.

5. Sanz M, Quirynen M; European Workshop in Periodontology Group A. Advances in the aetiology of periodontitis: Group A consensus report of the 5th European Workshop in Periodontology. J Clin Periodontol 2005;32(6 suppl):54–56.

6. Baker KA. The role of dental professionals and the patient in plaque control. Periodontol 2000 1995;8:108–113.

7. Sanz M, Teughels W; Group A of European Workshop on Periodontology. Innovations in non-surgical periodontal therapy: Consensus Report of the Sixth European Workshop on Periodontology. J Clin Periodontol 2008;35(8 suppl):3–7.

8. Linden G, Lyons A, Scannapieco FA. Periodontal systemic associations: Review of the evidence. J Clin Periodontol 2013;40:S8–S19.

9. American Academy of Periodontology. Comprehensive periodontal therapy: A statement by the American Academy of Periodontology. J Periodontol 2011;82:943–949.

10. Rethman MP, Harrel SK. Minimally invasive periodontal therapy: Will periodontal therapy remain a technologic laggard? J Periodontol 2010;81:1390–1395.

11. Drisko CH. Nonsurgical periodontal therapy. Periodontol 2000 2001;25:77–88.

12. Aimetti M. Nonsurgical periodontal treatment. Int J Esthet Dent 2014;9:251–267.

13. Poyato-Ferrera M, Segura-Egea JJ, Bullón-Fernández P. Comparison of modified Bass technique with normal toothbrushing practices for efficacy in supragingival plaque removal. Int J Dent Hyg 2003;1:110–114.

14. Rosema NA, Adam R, Grender JM, Van der Sluijs E, Supranoto SC, Van der Weijden GA. Gingival abrasion and recession in manual and oscillating-rotating power brush users. Int J Dent Hyg 2014;12:257–266.

15. Slot DE, Wiggelinkhuizen L, Rosema NA, Van der Weijden GA. The efficacy of manual toothbrushes following a brushing exercise: A systematic review. Int J Dent Hyg 2012;10:187–197.

16. Yaacob M, Worthington HV, Deacon SA, et al. Powered versus manual toothbrushing for oral health. Cochrane Database Syst Rev 2014;6:CD002281.

17. Dörfer CE, Staehle HJ, Wolff D. Three-year randomized study of manual and power toothbrush effects on pre-existing gingival recession. J Clin Periodontol 2016;43:512–519.

18. Chapple ILC, van der Weijden F, Doerfer C, et al. Primary prevention of periodontitis: Managing gingivitis. J Clin Periodontol 2015;42(suppl 16):S71–S76.

19. Tonetti MS, Pini-Prato G, Cortellini P. Periodontal regeneration of human intrabony defects. IV. Determinants of healing response. J Periodontol 1993;64:934–940.

20. Listgarten MA, Ellegaard B. Electron microscopic evidence of a cellular attachment between junctional epithelium and dental calculus. J Periodontal Res 1973;8:143–150.

21. Laleman I, Cortellini S, De Winter S, et al. Subgingival debridement: End points, methods and how often? Periodontol 2000 2017;75:189–204.

22. Nyman S, Westfelt E, Sarhed G, Karring T. Role of "diseased" root cementum in healing following treatment of periodontal disease. A clinical study. J Clin Periodontol 1988;15:464–468.

23. Nakib NM, Bissada NF, Simmelink JW, Goldstine SN. Endotoxin penetration into root cementum of periodontally healthy and diseased human teeth. J Periodontol 1982;53:368–378.

24. Tunkel J, Heinecke A, Flemmig TF. A systematic review of efficacy of machine-driven and manual subgingival debridement in the treatment of chronic periodontitis. J Clin Periodontol 2002;29(suppl 3):72–81.

25. Krishna R, De Stefano JA. Ultrasonic vs. hand instrumentation in periodontal therapy: Clinical outcomes. Periodontol 2000 2016;71:113–127.

26. Drisko CL. Periodontal debridement: Hand versus power driven scalers. Dent Hygiene News 1995;8:18–23.

27. Torfason T, Kiger R, Selvig KA, Egelberg J. Clinical improvement of gingival conditions following ultrasonic versus hand instrumentation of periodontal pockets. J Clin Periodontol 1979;6:165–176.

28. Benfenati MP, Montesani MT, Benfenati SP, Nathanson D. Scanning electron microscope: An SEM study of periodontally instrumented root surfaces, comparing sharp, dull, and damaged curettes and ultrasonic instruments. Int J Periodontics Restorative Dent 1987;2:50–67.

29. Vastardis S, Yukna RA, Rice DA, Mercante D. Root surface removal and resultant surface texture with diamond coated ultrasonic inserts: An in vitro and SEM study. J Clin Periodontol 2005;32:467–473.

30. Leon LE, Vogel RI. A comparison of the effectiveness of hand scaling and ultrasonic debridement in furcations as evaluated by differential dark-field microscopy. J Periodontol 1987;58:86–94.

31. Ruppert M, Cadosch J, Guindy J, Case D, Zappa U. In vivo ultrasonic debridement forces in bicuspids: A pilot study. J Periodontol 2002:73:418–422.

32. Walmsley AD, Lea SC, Landini G, Moses AJ. Advances in power driven pocket/root instrumentation. J Clin Periodontol 2008;35(8 suppl):22–28.

33. Smiley CJ, Tracy SL, Abt E, et al. Systematic review and meta-analysis on the nonsurgical treatment of chronic periodontitis by means of scaling and root planing with or without adjuncts. J Am Dent Assoc 2015;146:508–524.

34. John MT, Michalowicz BS, Kotsakis GA, Chu H. Network meta-analysis of studies included in the Clinical Practice Guideline on the nonsurgical treatment of chronic periodontitis. J Clin Periodontol 2017;44:603–611.

35. Aoki A, Sasaki KM, Watanabe H, Ishikawa I. Lasers in nonsurgical periodontal therapy. Periodontol 2000 2004;36:59–97.

36. Romanos GE, Henze M, Banihashemi S, Parsanejad HR, Winckler J, Nentwig GH. Removal of epithelium in periodontal pockets following diode (980 nm) laser application in the animal model: An in vitro study. Photomed Laser Surg 2004;22:177–183.

37. Cobb CM, Low SB, Coluzzi DJ. Lasers and the treatment of chronic periodontitis. Dent Clin North Am 2010;54:35–53.

38. Ishikawa I, Aoki A, Takasaki AA, Mizutani K, Sasaki KM, Izumi Y. Application of lasers in periodontics: True innovation or myth? Periodontol 2000 2009;50:90–126.

39. Folwaczny M, Aggstaller H, Mehl A, Hickel R. Removal of bacterial endotoxin from root surface with Er:YAG laser. Am J Dent 2003;16:3–5.

40. Schwarz F, Bieling K, Venghaus S, Sculean A, Jepsen S, Becker J. Influence of fluorescence-controlled Er:YAG laser radiation, the Vector system and hand instruments on periodontally diseased root surfaces in vivo. J Clin Periodontol 2006;33:200–208.

41. Soo L, Leichter JW, Windle J, et al. A comparison of Er:YAG laser and mechanical debridement for the non-surgical treatment of chronic periodontitis: A randomized, prospective clinical study. J Clin Periodontol 2012;39:537–545.

42. Sgolastra F, Petrucci A, Gatto R, Monaco A. Efficacy of Er:YAG laser in the treatment of chronic periodontitis: Systematic review and meta-analysis. Lasers Med Sci 2012;27:661–673.

43. Zhao Y, Yin Y, Tao L, Nie P, Tang Y, Zhu M. Er:YAG laser versus scaling and root planing as alternative or adjuvant for chronic periodontitis treatment: A systematic review. J Clin Periodontol 2014;41:1069–1079.

44. Mills MP, Rosen PS, Chambrone L, et al. American Academy of Periodontology best evidence consensus statement on the efficacy of laser therapy used alone or as an adjunct to non-surgical and surgical treatment of periodontitis and peri-implant diseases. J Periodontol 2018;89:737–742.

45. Allison RR, Moghissi K. Photodynamic therapy (PDT): PDT mechanisms. Clin Endosc 2013;46:24–29.

46. Fontana CR, Abernethy AD, Som S, et al. The antibacterial effect of photodynamic therapy in dental plaque-derived biofilms. J Periodontal Res 2009;44:751–759.

47. Azarpazhooh A, Shah P, Tenenbaum H, Goldberg M. The effect of photodynamic therapy for periodontitis: A systematic review and meta-analysis. J Periodontol 2010;81:4–14.

48. Atkinson DR, Cobb CM, Killoy WJ. The effect of an air-powder abrasive system on in vitro root surfaces. J Periodontol 1984;55:13–18.

49. Kontturi-Narhi V, Markkanen S, Markkanen H. Effects of airpolishing on dental plaque removal and hard tissues as evaluated by scanning electron microscopy. J Periodontol 1990;61:334–338.

50. Petersilka GJ. Subgingval air-polishing in the treatment of periodontal biofilm infection. Periodontol 2000 2011;55:124–142.

51. Sultan DA, Hill RG, Gillam DG. Air-polishing in subgingival root debridement: A critical literature review. J Dent Oral Biol 2017;2(10):1065.

52. Finlayson RS, Stevens FD. Subcutaneous facial emphysema secondary to use of the Cavi-Jet. J Periodontol 1988;59:315–317.

53. Sculean A, Bastendorf KD, Becker C, et al. A paradigm shift in mechanical biofilm management? Subgingival air polishing: A new way to improve mechanical biofilm management in the dental practice. Quintessence Int 2013;44:475–477.

54. Heitz-Mayfield LJA, Lang NP. Surgical and nonsurgical periodontal therapy. Learned and unlearned concepts. Periodontol 2000 2013;62:218–231.

55. Buchanan SA, Robertson PB. Calculus removal by scaling/root planing with and without surgical access. J Periodontol 1987;58:159–163.

56. Drisko CL. Periodontal debridement: Still the treatment of choice. J Evid Based Dent Pract 2014;(14 suppl):33–41.

57. Herrera D, Matesanz P, Bascones-Martínez A, Sanz M. Local and systemic antimicrobial therapy in periodontics. J Evid Based Dent Pract 2012;12(3 suppl):50–60.

58. Matesanz-Pérez P, García-Gargallo M, Figuero E, Bascones-Martínez A, Sanz M, Herrera D. A systematic review on the effects of local antimicrobials as adjuncts to subgingival debridement, compared with subgingival debridement alone, in the treatment of chronic periodontitis. J Clin Periodontol 2013;40:227–241.

59. Hanes PJ, Purvis JP. Local anti-infective therapy: Pharmacological agents. A systematic review. Ann Periodontol 2003;8:79–98.

60. Bonito AJ, Lux L, Lohr KN. Impact of local adjuncts to scaling and root planing in periodontal disease therapy: A systematic review. J Periodontol 2005;76:1227–1236.

61. Chambrone L, Vargas M, Arboleda S, et al. Efficacy of local and systemic antimicrobials in the non-surgical treatment of smokers with chronic periodontitis: A systematic review. J Periodontol 2016;87:1320–1332.

62. Rovai ES, Souto ML, Ganhito JA, Holzhausen M, Chambrone L, Pannuti CM. Efficacy of local antimicrobials in the non-surgical treatment of patients with periodontitis and diabetes: A systematic review. J Periodontol 2016;87:1406–1417.

63. Gunsolley JC. A meta-analysis of six-month studies of antiplaque and antigingivitis agents. J Am Dent Assoc 2006;137:1649–1657.

64. Hallmon WW, Rees TD. Local anti-infective therapy: Mechanical and physical approaches. A systematic review. Ann Periodontol 2003;8:99–114.

65. Cosyn J, Sabzevar MM. A systematic review on the effects of subgingival chlorhexidine gel administration in the treatment of chronic periodontitis. J Periodontol 2005;76:1805–1813.

66. Oosterwaal PJ, Mikx FH, Van 't Hof MA, Renggli HH. Short-term bactericidal activity of chlorhexidine gel, stannous fluoride gel and amine fluoride gel tested in periodontal pockets. J Clin Periodontol 1991;18:97–100.

67. Herrera D. Scaling and root planing is recommended in the nonsurgical treatment of chronic periodontitis. J Evid Based Dent Pract 2016;16:56–58.

68. van der Weijden GA, Timmerman MF. A systematic review of the clinical efficacy of subgingival debridement in the treatment of chronic periodontitis. J Clin Periodontol 2002;29(suppl 3):55–71.

69. Sigh J, Deshpande RN. Pathologic migration—Spontaneous correction following periodontal therapy: A case report. Quintessence Int 2002;33:65–68.

70. Quirynen M, Bollen CML, Vandekerckhove BN, Dekeyser C, Papaioannou W, Eyssen H. Full- vs. partial-mouth disinfection in the treatment of periodontal infections: Short-term clinical and microbiological observations. J Dent Res 1995;74:1459–1467.

71. Bollen CM, Mongardini C, Papaioannou W, van Steenberghe D, Quirynen M. The effect of a one-stage full-mouth disinfection on different intra-oral niches. Clinical and microbiological observations. J Clin Periodontol 1998;25:56–66.

72. Aimetti M, Romano F, Guzzi N, Carnevale G. One-stage full-mouth disinfection as a therapeutic approach for generalized aggressive periodontitis. J Periodontol 2011;82:845–853.

73. Aimetti M, Romano F, Guzzi N, Carnevale GF. Full-mouth disinfection and systemic antimicrobial therapy in generalized aggressive periodontitis: A randomized, placebo-controlled trial. J Clin Periodontol 2012;39:284–294.

74. Cobb CM. Non-surgical pocket therapy: Mechanical. Ann Periodontol 1996;1:443–490.

75. Hung HC, Douglass CW. Meta-analysis of the effect of scaling and root planing, surgical treatment and antibiotic therapies on periodontal probing depth and attachment loss. J Clin Periodontol 2002;29:975–986.

76. Lindhe J, Nyman S, Westfelt E, Socransky SS, Haffajee A. Critical probing depths in periodontal therapy. Compend Contin Educ Dent 1982;3:421–430.

77. Ehnevid H, Jansson LE. Effects of furcation involvements on periodontal status and healing in adjacent proximal sites. J Periodontol 2001;72:871–876.

78. Lang NP, Bartold PM. Periodontal health. J Clin Periodontol 2018;45(suppl 20):S9–S16.

79. Lang NP, Adler R, Joss A, Nyman S. Absence of bleeding on probing. An indicator of periodontal stability. J Clin Periodontol 1990;17:714–721.

80. Matuliene G, Pjetursson BE, Salvi GE, et al. Influence of residual pockets on progression of periodontitis and tooth loss: Results after 11 years of maintenance. J Clin Periodontol 2008;35:685–695.

81. Badersten A, Nilvéus R, Egelberg J. Scores of plaque, bleeding, suppuration and probing depth to predict probing attachment loss. 5 years of observation following nonsurgical periodontal therapy. J Clin Periodontol 1990;17:102–107.

82. Schätzle M, Löe H, Bürgin W, Ånerud Å, Boysen H, Lang NP. Clinical course of chronic periodontitis. J Clin Periodontol 2003;30:887–901.

83. Schätzle M, Löe H, Lang NP, Bürgin W, Ånerud Å, Boysen H. The clinical course of chronic periodontitis: IV. Gingival inflammation as a risk factor for tooth mortality. J Clin Periodontol 2004;31:1122–1127.

84. Sanz I, Alonso B, Carasol M, Herrera D, Sanz M. Nonsurgical treatment of periodontitis. J Evid Base Dent Pract 2012;12(3 suppl):76–88.

85. Wennström JL, Tomasi C, Bertelle A, Dellasega E. Full-mouth ultrasonic debridement versus quadrant scaling and root planing as an initial approach in the treatment of chronic periodontitis. J Clin Periodontol 2005;32:851–859.

86. Rabbani GM, Ash MM Jr, Caffesse RG. The effectiveness of subgingival scaling and root planing in calculus removal. J Periodontol 1981;52:119–123.

87. Waerhaug J. Healing of the dento-epithelial junction following sub gingival plaque control. II: As observed on extracted teeth. J Periodontol 1978;49:119–134.

88. Loos B, Nylund K, Claffey N, Egelberg J. Clinical effects of root debridement in molar and non-molar teeth. A 2-year follow up. J Clin Periodontol 1989;16:498–504.

89. Tomasi C, Leyland AH, Wennström JL. Factors influencing the outcome of non-surgical periodontal treatment: A multilevel approach. J Clin Periodontol 2007;34:682–690.

90. Gerber FA, Sahrmann P, Schmidlin OA, Heumann C, Beer JH, Schmidlin PR. Influence of obesity on the outcome of non-surgical periodontal therapy: A systematic review. BMC Oral Health 2016;16:90–110.

91. Segelnick SL, Wienberg MA. Reevaluation of initial therapy: When is the appropriate time? J Periodontal 2006;77:1598–1601.

92. Badersten A, Nilveus R, Egelberg J. Effect of non-surgical periodontal therapy. II. Severely advanced periodontitis. J Clin Periodontol 1984;11:63–76.

93. Nibali L, Pelekos G, Onabolu O, Donos N. Effect and timing of non-surgical treatment prior to periodontal regeneration: A systematic review. Clin Oral Investig 2015;19:1755–1761.

94. Trombelli L, Simonelli A, Minenna L, Vecchiatini R, Farina R. Simplified procedures to treat periodontal intraosseous defects in esthetic areas. Periodontol 2000 2018;77:93–110.

95. Ribeiro FV, Casarin RCV, Palma MA, Júnior FH, Sallum EA, Casati MZ. Clinical and patient-centered outcomes after minimally invasive non-surgical or surgical approaches for the treatment of intrabony defects: A randomized clinical trial. J Periodontol 2011;82:1256–1266.

96. Ribeiro FV, Casarin RC, Palma MA, Júnior FH, Sallum EA, Casati MZ. Clinical and microbiological changes after minimally invasive therapeutic approaches in intrabony defects: A 12-month follow-up. Clin Oral Investig 2013;17:1635–1644.

97. Nibali L, Pometti D, Chen TT, Tu YK. Minimally invasive non-surgical approach for the treatment of periodontal intrabony defects: A retrospective analysis. J Clin Periodontol 2015;42:853–859.

98. Aimetti M, Ferrarotti F, Mariani GM, Romano F. A novel flapless approach versus minimally invasive surgery in periodontal regeneration with enamel matrix derivative proteins: A 24-month randomized controlled clinical trial. Clin Oral Investig 2017;21:327–337.

99. Nibali L, Yeh YC, Pometti D, Tu YK. Long-term stability of intrabony defects treated with minimally invasive non-surgical therapy. J Clin Periodontol 2018;45:1458–1464.

100. Tonetti MS, Prato GP, Cortellini P. Factors affecting the healing response of intrabony defects following guided tissue regeneration and access flap surgery. J Clin Periodontol 1996;23:548–556.

101. Wikesjö UM, Nilvéus RE, Selvig KA. Significance of early wound healing on periodontal repair: A review. J Periodontol 1992;63:158–165.

102. Haney JM, Nilvéus RE, McMillan PJ, Wikesjö UM. Periodontal repair in dogs: Expanded polytetrafluoroethylene barrier membranes support wound stabilization and enhance bone regeneration. J Periodontol 1993;64:883–890.

103. Nibali L, Pometti D, Tu YK, Donos N. Clinical and radiographic outcomes following non-surgical therapy of periodontal infrabony defects: A retrospective study. J Clinical Periodontol 2011;38:50–57.

104. Hancock EB. Regeneration procedures. In: American Academy of Periodontology. Proceedings of the World Workshop on Clinical Periodontics. American Academy of Periodontology, 1989:11–13.

105. Stahl SS, Froum S. Human intrabony lesion responses to debridement, porous hydroxyapatite implants and teflon barrier membranes. 7 histologic case reports. J Clin Periodontol 1991;18:605–610.

106. Wikesjö UM, Nilvéus RE. Periodontal repair in dogs: Effect of wound stabilization on healing. J Periodontol 1990;61:719–724.

107. Dragoo M. Regeneration of the Periodontal Attachment in Humans. Philadelphia: Lea & Febiger, 1981.

108. Wilson TG Jr, Carnio J, Schenk R, Myers G. Absence of histological signs of chronic inflammation following closed subgingival scaling and root planing using the dental endoscope: Human biopsies – A pilot study. J Periodontol 2008;79:2036–2041.

109. Aimetti M, Ferrarotti F, Mariani GM, Fratini A, Giraudi M, Romano F. Enamel matrix derivative proteins in combination with flapless approach for periodontal regeneration of infrabony defects: A 2-year prospective case series. Int J Periodontics Restorative Dent 2016;36:797–805.

110. Bosshardt DD. Biological mediators and periodontal regeneration: A review of enamel matrix proteins at the cellular and molecular levels. J Clin Periodontol 2008;35(8 suppl):87–105.

111. Hammarström L, Heijl L, Gestrelius S. Periodontal regeneration in a buccal dehiscence model in monkeys after application of enamel matrix proteins. J Clin Periodontol 1997;24:669–677.

112. Miron RJ, Sculean A, Cochran DL, et al. Twenty years of enamel matrix derivative: The past, the present and the future. J Clin Periodontol 2016;43:668–683.

113. Venezia E, Goldstein M, Boyan BD, Schwartz Z. The use of enamel matrix derivative in the treatment of periodontal defects: A literature review and meta-analysis. Crit Rev Oral Biol Med 2004;15:382–402.

114. Esposito M, Grusovin MG, Papanikolau N, Coulthard P, Worthington HV. Enamel matrix derivative (Emdogain®) for periodontal tissue regeneration in intrabony defects. Cochrane Database Syst Rev 2009;4:CD003875.

115. Koop R, Merheb J, Quirynen M. Periodontal regeneration with enamel matrix derivative in reconstructive periodontal therapy: A systematic review. J Periodontol 2012;83:707–720.

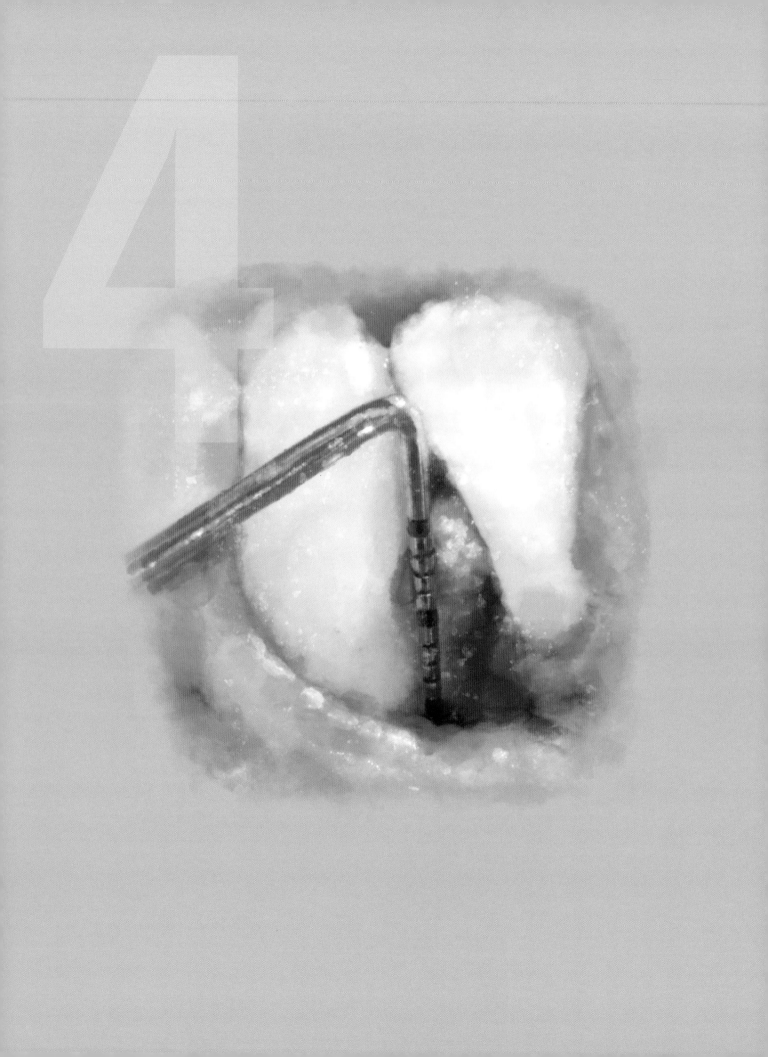

SIMPLIFIED SURGICAL REGENERATIVE PROCEDURES: THE SINGLE-FLAP APPROACH

Leonardo Trombelli, DDS, PhD
Roberto Farina, DDS, PhD, MSc
Anna Simonelli, DDS, PhD

SURGICAL TREATMENT OF INTRAOSSEOUS DEFECTS

Indications for surgery

Although nonsurgical treatment may result in a substantial improvement of the clinical conditions of the lesion (as illustrated in chapter 3), surgical access of the defect may be required in the following situations:

- A residual deep (ie, ≥ 6-mm) bleeding pocket associated with a radiographic angular defect
- Presence of a concomitant root abnormality, including enamel pearl/projection (Fig 4-1) and cemental tear (Fig 4-2)
- Presence of a concomitant degree II or III interradicular lesion

Although substantial clinical improvements can be achieved by treating intrabony defects with surgical regenerative treatment, clinical trials have consistently reported a great variability in outcomes. This suggests that many factors may be responsible for the end results of treatment, including socioeconomic background, form of periodontal disease, persistence of specific pathogens, differences in clinical experience, and surgical skill and clinical experience of the clinicians.[1] The main sources of clinical variability are the patient, the defect, and technical (surgery-associated) factors.[2] Therefore, a careful selection of patients and defects as well as proper technical competence with the surgical technique are paramount to improve the prognosis of a regenerative procedure.

When considering patient characteristics that may affect the regenerative outcome, available evidence indicates that the persistence of poor self-performed plaque control,

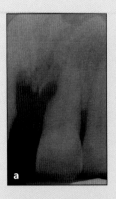
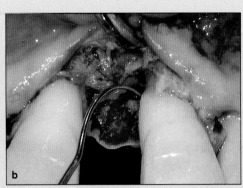

Fig 4-1 Presence of an enamel projection on the root surface of a maxillary central incisor. *(a)* Radiographic appearance. *(b)* Intraoperative view.

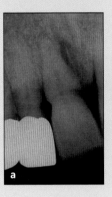
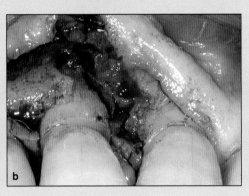

Fig 4-2 Cemental tear at the mesial aspect of the root surface in a maxillary central incisor. *(a)* Radiographic appearance. *(b)* Intraoperative view.

high levels of bleeding on probing (BOP) in the dentition, and the persistence of high total bacterial loads or of specific microbial pathogens have all been associated with poor clinical outcomes.[1] These findings reinforce the need for the following:

- *Treatment for periodontal inflammation.* Effective nonsurgical periodontal treatment based on multiple sessions of supra- and subgingival debridement can substantially reduce the level of periodontal infection and inflammation (BOP < 20%).
- *Oral hygiene.* The patient should be adequately motivated to perform oral hygiene measures to reach the proper level of supragingival plaque control (full-mouth plaque score < 15%).
- *Timing of the surgical treatment planning.* The surgical regenerative procedure should be preceded by the surgical correction of other periodontally compromised areas of the dentition. This way, the regeneration process will occur when the overall periodontal bacterial load is relevantly reduced.
- *Preventive protocol.* A stringent secondary preventive protocol based on routine, professional mechanical plaque removal,[3] as well as repeated oral hygiene instruction, is necessary to ensure short- and long-term regenerative outcomes.

A consistent amount of data showed that regenerative outcomes (ie, clinical attachment, bone gain) following regenerative procedures are affected by cigarette smoking. Patients who smoke showed significantly impaired regenerative outcomes compared with nonsmokers, especially for guided tissue regeneration (GTR).[4–10] Thus, smoking cessation programs should be recommended to prevent periodontitis recurrence and to ensure the long-term stability of the attachment gain.

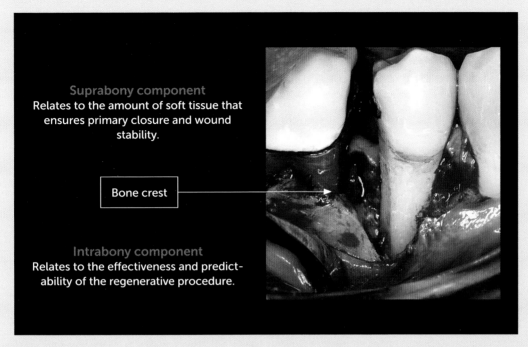

Fig 4-3 Suprabony and intrabony components of an intraosseous defect. The suprabony component relates to the amount of soft tissue that ensures primary closure and wound stability. The intrabony component relates to the effectiveness and predictability of the regenerative procedure.

When considering a periodontal intraosseous defect, two different components may be identified in relation to the bone crest (Fig 4-3):

• *Suprabony component.* This extends approximately from 2 mm apical to the cemento enamel junction to the bone crest. This component is related to the amount of soft tissue that ensures primary closure and wound stability after regenerative periodontal treatment.
• *Intrabony component.* This extends from the bone crest to the base of the defect. The severity of this component strongly affects tooth prognosis but may be reduced or completely filled through periodontal reconstructive treatments.

Periodontal intraosseous defects have been classified according to their morphology (ie, number of residual bony walls), width of the defect, radiographic angle, and severity (ie, depth of the defect). With respect to the residual alveolar bony walls, intraosseous defects are commonly classified as three-wall, two-wall, and one-wall defects (Fig 4-4). However, in relation to the anatomy of the supporting bone combined with the biofilm-induced periodontal inflammatory process, a more complex defect morphology is frequently identified, usually with a three-wall component in the most apical portion of the defect and two- and/or one-wall components in the most coronal portions (Fig 4-5). The width of the intraosseous defect may be assessed in radiographs by the angle between the root surface and a line from the most apical point of the intraosseous defect to its most coronal margin[3,9–11] (Fig 4-6); the depth of the defect can be accurately evaluated by probing bone level (Fig 4-7).

The characteristics of the defect, such as the width of the intrabony component, the defect angle, and the residual bony walls, have been shown to substantially affect the regenerative

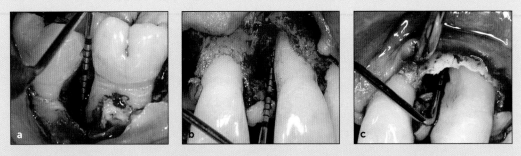

Fig 4-4 Paradigmatic cases of mainly *(a)* one-wall, *(b)* two-wall, and *(c)* three-wall intraosseous defects.

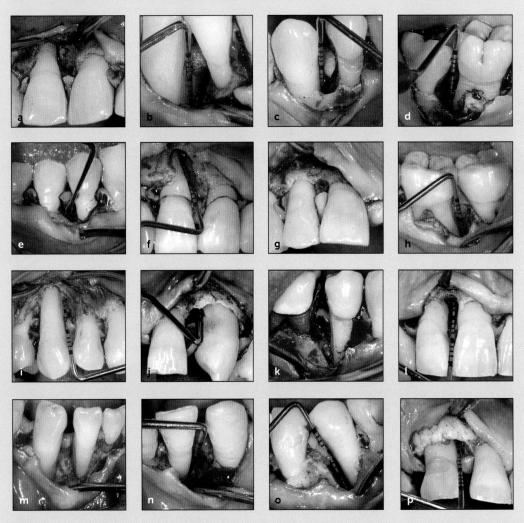

Fig 4-5 *(a to p)* Defects showing different soft and hard tissue morphologic characteristics that can be accessed by the single-flap approach.

outcome. In this respect, deeper defects with wider defect angle and/or greater one-wall component are associated with a poorer prognosis of the regenerative procedure (Fig 4-8). The features of the defect affect the regenerative outcome for several reasons:

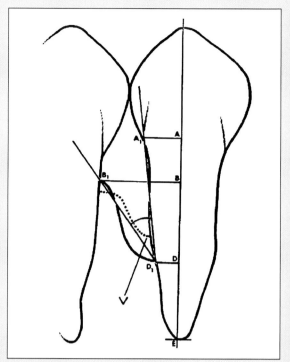

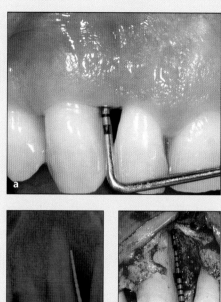

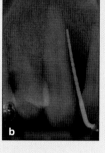

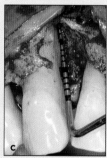

Fig 4-6 Identification of defect angle.[11] The defect angle is defined by two lines. The first line is constructed along the root surface from D_l, the most apical part of the defect, to A_l. The second line follows the defect surface from D_l to B_l, the most coronal part of the defect where it touches the neighboring tooth.

Fig 4-7 (a to c) Clinical, radiographic, and intrasurgical evaluation of defect depth by probing (courtesy of Dr Luigi Minenna).

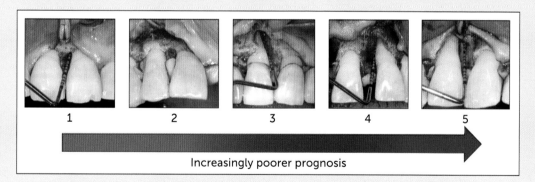

Increasingly poorer prognosis

Fig 4-8 Intraosseous defects with different prognoses to regenerative treatment. From 1 to 5, the depth and width of the lesion as well as the defect angle increase, whereas the number of residual bony walls decreases, thus challenging the treatment outcome.

- The inherent regenerative potential of the lesion. The characteristics of the lesion affect the amount of stem/progenitor cells involved in the regenerative process.
- The capability of the defect morphology to ensure blood clot stability. This is a prerequisite for tissue regeneration.
- The biomechanical support provided by the defect configuration to the surgical flap.

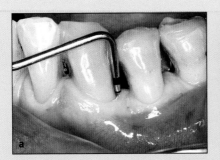 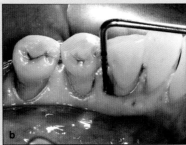 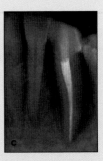

Fig 4-9 Treatment of a periodontal intraosseous defect with a buccal single-flap approach plus GTR. *(a and b)* Presurgical probing depth (PD) and clinical attachment level (CAL) loss at distobuccal and distolingual aspects of a mandibular first premolar. Class II mobility was detected before surgery, so the tooth was splinted. *(c)* Preoperative radiographic view of the lesion. Because of the negative response of the tooth to the pulp vitality test, endodontic treatment was performed prior to periodontal regenerative surgery.   →

Because of this, the clinician should consider regenerative devices and proper flap design. Specific regenerative devices (eg, titanium-reinforced membrane, additional graft biomaterials, biologic agents) can enhance the conditions for space provision, blood clot stability, and soft tissue support. This can help to compensate for the challenges of certain intraosseous defects, such as those with a wider angle or fewer bony walls. In addition, choosing the most appropriate flap design can greatly help to achieve and maintain wound stability, thus reducing the detrimental effects of the defect morphology.

The endodontic status of the tooth should be properly diagnosed prior to the regenerative procedure because a concomitant endodontic infection may heavily impact the outcome. A proper root canal treatment does not seem to negatively affect the healing response and the long-term stability of deep intrabony defects treated with GTR[12] (Fig 4-9). When approaching a regenerative surgical procedure, treatment planning should consider the following aspects:

- Careful assessment of tooth vitality and root canal treatment during the cause-related phase of the periodontal therapy. Nonvital teeth must receive root canal therapy, and any inadequate endodontic treatments should be redone.
- Teeth where the intraosseous lesion extends at the root apex can be preventively endodontically treated.[13]
- Necessary endodontic treatment or retreatment should be performed well in advance of the regenerative surgery (eg, 4 to 6 months beforehand).

Another factor that needs be considered before regenerative procedures is mobility of the tooth. An excessive jiggling movement may greatly affect wound stability, which in turn would compromise periodontal regeneration.[14] A limited presurgery mobility (< 1 mm horizontally) is compatible with successful regenerative treatment.[14] These observations lead to the following clinical recommendations:

- Presence of secondary occlusal trauma on the tooth candidate for regeneration should be assessed, and occlusal adjustment must be performed as needed during the nonsurgical phase of treatment. The need for a bite guard should also be considered (Fig 4-10).

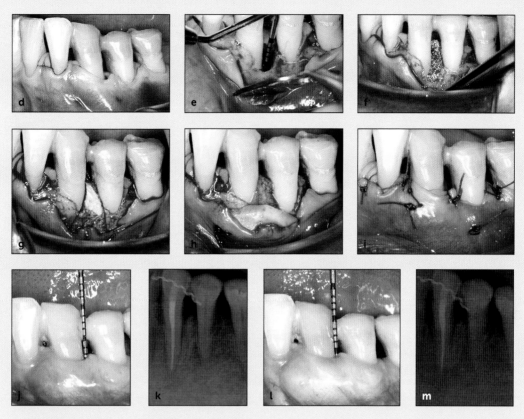

Fig 4-9 (cont) *(d)* The flap was designed according to the single-flap approach principles. *(e)* Intrasurgical assessment of the supraosseous and intraosseous components of the defect. The defect was predominantly a three-wall defect. *(f)* The defect was grafted with hydroxyapatite (HA) material (Biostite, Gaba Vebas). *(g)* A resorbable collagen membrane (Paroguide, Gaba Vebas) was used to cover the defect. *(h)* A connective tissue graft harvested from a maxillary edentulous area was fixed to the flap using internal mattress sutures. *(i)* The buccal flap was repositioned and sutured. *(j)* Soft tissue healing at 12 months following surgery. *(k)* Radiographic view of the treated site at 12 months. *(l)* Probing measurements and *(m)* radiographic view at 8 years, showing the stable conditions of the regenerated periodontal support.

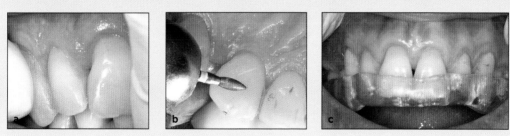

Fig 4-10 *(a)* Presurgical mobility (grade 1) with fremitus of a maxillary canine with a deep intraosseous periodontal defect. *(b)* An occlusal adjustment was performed before regenerative treatment. *(c)* A bite guard was provided.

- Teeth with a horizontal mobility greater than 1 mm should be splinted before or immediately following the surgical procedure[14,15] (Fig 4-11; see also Fig 4-9).
- Tooth mobility should be monitored during the healing phase, and any increase in mobility should be detected and managed appropriately.[1]
- The decision whether to maintain or remove the splint should be made at the completion of tissue maturation phase (at least 12 months after surgery).

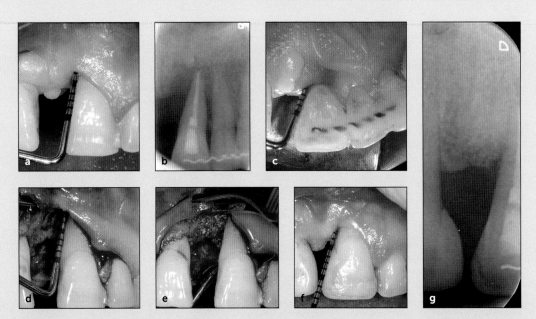

Fig 4-11 Regenerative treatment of a deep periodontal intraosseous defect. Clinical *(a)* and radiographic *(b)* views. *(c)* Due to tooth hypermobility, intracoronal splinting was performed before surgery. *(d)* Clinical appearance at the completion of intrasurgical debridement. *(e)* Deproteinized bovine bone mineral (DBBM) conditioned by enamel matrix derivative (EMD) was positioned to fill the intrabony component of the defect. *(f and g)* Clinical and radiographic condition at 4 years after surgery. The intracoronal splint is still in position.

Technical factors for successful regenerative treatment

When considering the technical aspects of periodontal regenerative procedures for intraosseous defects, four major factors seem to be most essential for a successful outcome: elimination of biofilm, flap design and suturing technique, regenerative technology, and minimization of soft tissue recession.

First, the dental biofilm must be eliminated from the area of the root surface that has been left contaminated by previous nonsurgical treatment. In this respect, surgical access must be planned on the defect morphology to provide optimal conditions for mechanical plaque removal and root conditioning as well as removal of the granulation tissue (Fig 4-12).

Secondly, flap design and suturing technique should be chosen to reduce the chances of postsurgical infection and contamination of the blood clot and the implanted biomaterial or biologic agent. Even if there is an apparent tissue approximation at the time of the surgical closure, postsurgical shrinkage of the soft tissues during the early healing phase often results in substantial exposure of the graft and/or membrane. This can lead to bacterial contamination of the wound, jeopardizing the process of biologic events leading to periodontal regeneration (Fig 4-13). Moreover, when autogenous bone chips or bone-substitute particles are used, incomplete tissue coverage may lead to the immediate, partial, or complete exfoliation of the implanted graft. Loss of primary closure in the interdental area often results in interdental soft tissue craters, making it difficult for the clinician and the patient to perform adequate plaque control during the healing phase.

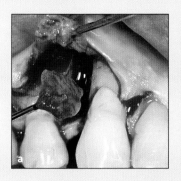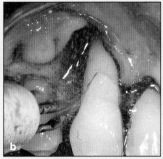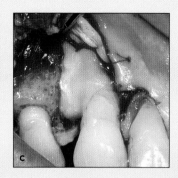

Fig 4-12 *(a)* The granulation tissue filling the intraosseous defect was removed using manual instruments (Hirschfeld file scaler, Hu-Friedy). *(b)* Intrasurgical root debridement was performed using both manual and ultrasonic instruments. *(c)* The root surface was conditioned with 24% ethylenediaminetetraacetic acid (EDTA) gel for 2 minutes to remove the smear layer.

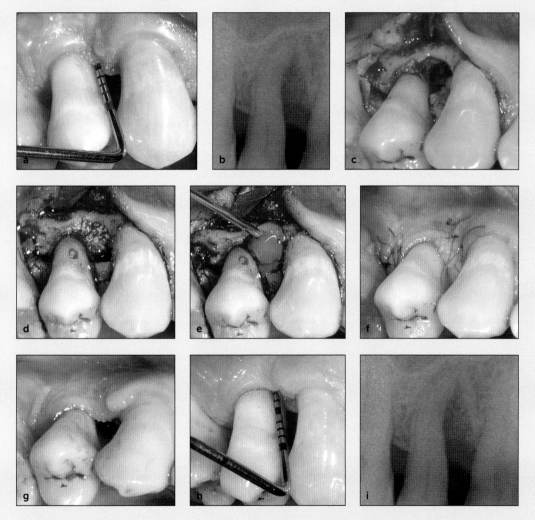

Fig 4-13 *(a and b)* Preoperative CAL loss and bone loss at the mesial aspect of a maxillary first premolar. *(c)* Intraosseous defect at the completion of intrasurgical debridement. *(d)* Particles of DBBM conditioned by EMD were positioned to fill the intrabony component of the defect. *(e)* EMD was injected to cover the grafted DBBM particles and condition the portion of the root surface coronal to the bone crest. *(f)* Primary intention healing was obtained with a horizontal internal mattress suture at the base of the papilla and an additional internal mattress suture at the most coronal portion of the papilla. *(g)* Early wound dehiscence at 2 weeks after surgery. *(h)* Persistent 7-mm pocket at 6 months after surgery. *(i)* Incomplete defect remineralization at 6 months after surgery.

The third factor is the selection of the appropriate regenerative technology. This should be related to the severity and morphology of the defect and informed by the desired treatment outcome. The regenerative device should be synergistically matched to the flap design.

The fourth factor is to minimize postsurgical soft tissue recession on both the interproximal and buccal aspects of the treated tooth, which would compromise the preexisting esthetic appearance (Fig 4-14). In analyzing the prevalence distribution of intraosseous defects with respect to tooth type, a considerable proportion of lesions involve teeth in the most esthetically sensitive area.[16] In addition to esthetic impairment, loss of the interdental papilla may also create problems relating to phonetics and food impaction.

Flap design and suturing technique

Historical surgical approaches chosen to access and treat periodontal intraosseous defects were based on flap designs characterized by either minimal soft tissue resection[17,18] or total preservation of interdental tissues, such as the papilla preservation technique (PPT)[19] and its variants.[20–24] All these flap designs are based on the elevation of a double mucoperiosteal flap involving both the buccal and lingual/palatal aspects.

While primary closure may be easily achieved when the periodontal defect is located on the buccal aspect of the tooth, as in dehiscence-type defects or interradicular lesions, primary closure in the interdental area often represents a challenge for the clinician. When conventional access flap surgery has been associated with reconstructive procedures—namely GTR—it has been reported that lack of primary closure of the interdental space, flap dehiscence, or membrane exposure occurs in 70% to 80% of the treated sites.[8,25–27] In response to this, new surgical techniques have been specifically designed and developed to optimize functional and esthetic outcomes of reconstructive procedures in the interdental area.[19,20,22,23,28]

From a clinical standpoint, the factors that improve predictability of regenerative procedures are *(1)* surgical flap design and management and *(2)* suturing technique.

The design and management of the flap should be chosen for best flap survival and graft coverage. The supracrestal soft tissues must be preserved as much as possible, primary closure must be obtained in the interdental area, and postoperative shrinkage of the papilla should be minimized. The suturing technique must be chosen to optimize primary closure and thus ensure the primary conditions for blood clot stabilization and maturation in a biologic environment. The wound should be protected from biomechanical and microbiologic challenges.

Technical options for the selection of flap design and suturing technique for regenerative procedures in intraosseous defects have been extensively revised and include the following:

- Papilla preservation technique[19]
- Interproximal tissue maintenance[20]
- Modified and simplified papilla preservation techniques[22,23]
- Single-flap approach[29]

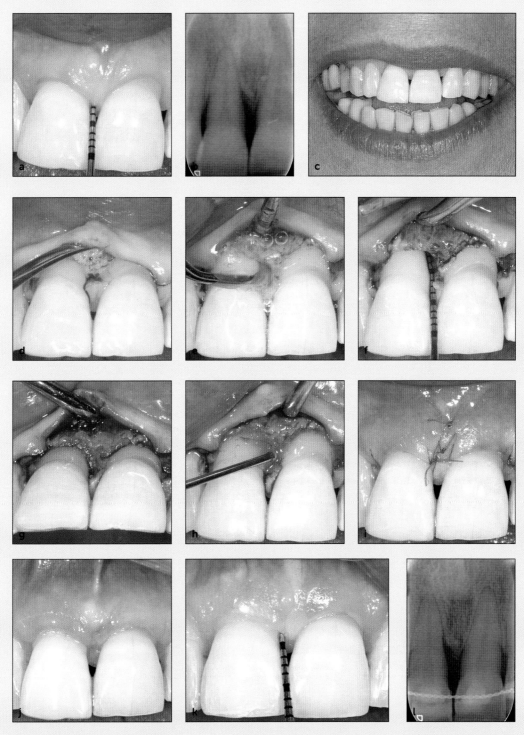

Fig 4-14 *(a)* Treatment of a maxillary central incisor with a preoperative PD of 7 mm. *(b)* Radiographic view before surgery. *(c)* Note the amount of exposed interdental papillae during the smile. This patient has a high esthetic demand. *(d)* The intraosseous defect is accessed by the single-flap approach. *(e)* Intrasurgical debridement of the defect with ultrasonic instruments. *(f)* The defect is characterized by a narrow angle and a 5-mm-deep intraosseous component. *(g)* Following a first application of EMD, the intraosseous component of the lesion is filled with DBBM with the bioactive agent. *(h)* Application of second layer of EMD. *(i)* Wound closure is obtained with two internal mattress sutures and additional interrupted sutures. *(j)* At 2 weeks following surgery, complete flap closure is evident. *(k)* Clinical view 5 years after surgery. *(l)* Radiographic view 5 years after surgery.

The flap design may be classified according to the following:

- The outline of the incision, which affects the preservation of the interdental supracrestal soft tissues.
- The elevation of either a single (buccal or lingual/palatal) or a double (buccal and lingual/palatal) flap in relation to the surgical trauma exerted at the interproximal soft tissues.

Flap designs that preserve the integrity of the interdental supracrestal soft tissue by elevating a double flap include the PPT introduced by Takei et al[19] and its subsequent surgical variants such as the interproximal tissue maintenance (ITM) technique,[20] the modified papilla preservation technique (MPPT)[22] (Fig 4-15), and the simplified papilla preservation technique (SPPT)[23] (Video 4-1).

All of these flap designs are characterized by the fact that no incisions are made through the interdental papilla. Either the buccal or the lingual/palatal papilla is therefore included in the contralateral lingual/palatal or buccal flap, respectively, leaving the volume of the supracrestal soft tissues intact in the interproximal area. The application of this concept as MPPT for GTR treatment of deep intraosseous defects resulted in 73% to 80% of complete coverage of the membrane during the healing phase.[4,30] A study performed by Cortellini et al[4] showed that MPPT in association with a titanium-reinforced expanded polytetrafluoroethylene (ePTFE) membrane determined a significantly greater clinical attachment level (CAL) gain compared with a conventional (ie, modified Widman flap) approach with or without a standard ePTFE membrane. When SPPT was used for GTR with resorbable membranes, this approach consistently resulted in 46% to 67% of complete membrane coverage during healing.[14] PPT, MPPT, and ITM techniques place the incision line away from the bone defect, thus limiting graft or membrane exposure during postsurgical healing. In addition, MPPT includes a coronal displacement of the buccal flap, which greatly contributes to primary closure over the graft or membrane and may result in CAL gain coronal to the alveolar crest.[22]

When compared with conventional access flap surgery, papilla preservation techniques showed greater amounts of CAL gain, showing that the healing of a flap that provides primary intention healing and greater wound stability may result in better outcomes. This outcome was underlined by several authors: Graziani et al[31] showed that conservative surgery based on papilla preservation techniques results in 2.48 mm of CAL gain 1 year after surgery compared with 1.57 mm with conservative surgery based on conventional access surgery. Moreover, Tu et al[32] give an indirect support to this thesis with a systematic review assessing the temporal trend of healing of surgical flaps used for intrabony defects. Data showed a consistent increase of access flap performance over a 15-year period. This temporal trend can be interpreted as the result of the more widespread usage of papilla preservation flaps in more recent years.

Specific suturing techniques are described depending on the selected flap design; however, when suturing for a regenerative procedure, the following general recommendations are indicated:

- Use 5-0 to 7-0 sutures, depending on the thickness of the tissue to be sutured.
- Leave the sutures in place for at least 14 days. This provides flap adaptation and closure until there is sufficient maturation of the wound to resist any disruptive mechanical forces acting on the wound margins.

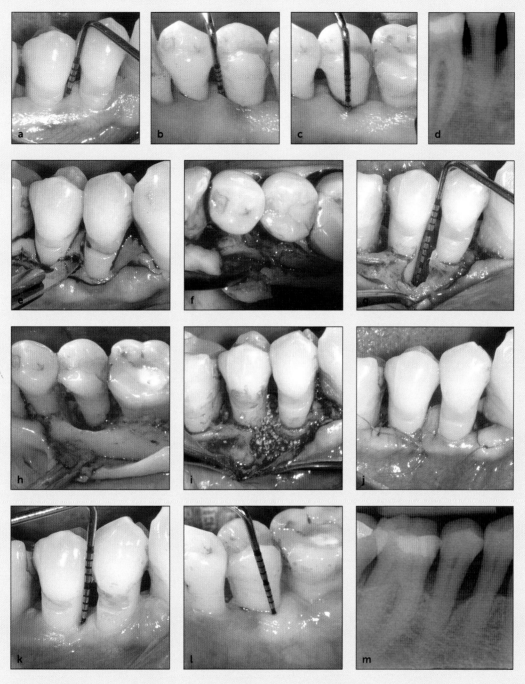

Fig 4-15 Treatment of a periodontal intraosseous defect with a double-flap approach (MPPT).[22] *(a to c)* Preoperative PD and CAL loss at the mesiobuccal, mesiolingual, and lingual aspects of a mandibular second premolar. The defects presented a buccal and lingual extension. *(d)* Radiograph of the lesion before surgery. *(e)* Sulcular incisions were made following the gingival margin of teeth included in the surgical area. An incision was made at the buccal aspect of the interdental papilla overlying the intraosseous defect according to the MPPT. *(f)* A microsurgical periosteal elevator was used to raise a flap on both the buccal and lingual sides. *(g)* The buccal aspect of the intraosseous defect after surgical debridement. The intrabony component was 7 mm deep. *(h)* Lingual aspect of the intraosseous defect after surgical debridement. *(i)* The intraosseous component of the defect was filled with DBBM mixed with EMD. *(j)* Primary closure was achieved according to the MPPT suturing technique. The papilla between the canine and first premolar was apically positioned for pocket elimination. *(k to m)* Interproximal and lingual probing depths and radiograph view at the 5-year follow-up.

- Place the sutures in the interdental area overlying the intraosseous defect coronal to the mucogingival junction (ie, in the keratinized gingiva) to ensure proper flap stability.
- Ensure closure of passively adapted flaps. Sutures should not be tied too tightly or exert excessive tension on the flap.
- Use internal mattress sutures to coronally advance the flaps without tension on the flap edges. Interrupted sutures may be used to approximate wound margins and close releasing incisions.
- Limit (or avoid) the use of conventional interrupted loop sutures or external cross-mattress sutures to close the flap overlying the intraosseous defect. Although cross-mattress sutures may result in optimal flap closure without having suture material in direct contact with the graft biomaterial, they tend to flatten the interdental papillae, particularly in thin-scalloped biotypes.
- Suture the vertical releasing incision using interrupted sutures placed in an apicocoronal direction to maximize the tension-free coronal displacement of the flap.

Anatomical characteristics informing flap design

Anatomical characteristics related to the area of the dentition to be treated, patient biotype, and defect morphology should be carefully evaluated because they will influence the selection of the flap design. These include the following[5,20,22,23,29]:

- Mesiodistal dimension (width) of the interdental space
- Distance from the tip of the papilla to the underlying bone crest in the interdental area (ie, apicocoronal dimension of the supracrestal soft tissues)
- Apicocoronal amount of keratinized tissue
- Periodontal biotype of the patient
- Type of tooth presenting with the intraosseous defect
- Buccolingual extension of the intraosseous defect (see Table 4-1)

INDICATIONS AND ADVANTAGES FOR THE SINGLE-FLAP APPROACH

What is the single-flap approach?

In 2007, the authors proposed the first simplified surgical procedure to access the intraosseous lesion for regenerative purposes.[29] This procedure, defined as the *single-flap approach* (SFA), is based on the elevation of a flap on one aspect (ie, buccal or lingual/palatal) only, thus preserving the integrity of the interdental soft tissue. The main surgical characteristics of the SFA can be summarized as follows (Fig 4-16)[33]:

- Envelope flap with limited mesiodistal extension (although the primary incision should be extended mesiodistally to provide adequate surgical access with no excessive tension on the flap)

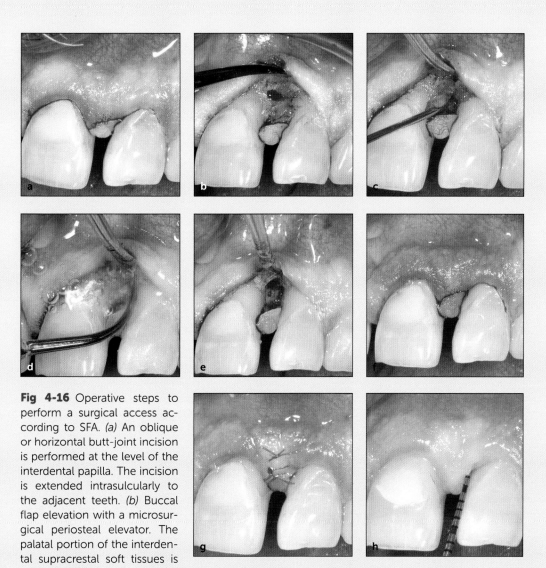

Fig 4-16 Operative steps to perform a surgical access according to SFA. *(a)* An oblique or horizontal butt-joint incision is performed at the level of the interdental papilla. The incision is extended intrasulcularly to the adjacent teeth. *(b)* Buccal flap elevation with a microsurgical periosteal elevator. The palatal portion of the interdental supracrestal soft tissues is left undetached. *(c)* Intrasurgical debridement with hand instruments (Hirschfeld file scaler). *(d)* Intrasurgical debridement with ultrasonic instruments with ultrathin perio tip. *(e)* Intraoperative view of the debrided root surface and degranulated defect. *(f)* Passive adaptation of the flap to its original position. *(g)* Would closure is obtained with a first horizontal internal mattress suture at the base of the papilla and a second internal mattress suture at the most coronal portion of the papilla. *(h)* Clinical view at 1 year after surgery, showing the CAL gain and the maintained gingival contour. (Reprinted with permission from Trombelli et al.[33])

- Elevation of a full-thickness flap only on either the buccal (more frequently) or lingual/palatal aspect depending on defect extension/morphology as diagnosed by bone sounding (see pages 103 to 104)
- Interproximal supracrestal soft tissues are left intact and undetached at the opposite side
- One-side surgical access must warrant proper root/defect debridement

Table 4-1 Clinical indications for each surgical option

	PPT	ITM	MPPT	SPPT	SFA
Width of interdental space	Wide	Wide	Wide	Wide/narrow	Wide/narrow
Apicocoronal dimension of the supracrestal soft tissues	Large	Large	Large	Large/small	Large/small
Apicocoronal amount of keratinized tissue	Large (for buccal incision only)/ small	Large/small	Large	Large/small	Large/small
Vestibule depth	Shallow/deep (for buccal incision only)	Shallow/deep	Deep	Shallow/deep	Shallow/deep
Frenum insertion	High (for buccal incision only)/ low	High/low	High	High/low	High/low
Gingival phenotype	Thick-flat (for buccal incision only)/ thin-scalloped	Thick-flat/ thin-scalloped	Thick-flat	Thick-flat/ thin-scalloped	Thick-flat/ thin-scalloped
Location of the intraosseous defect (tooth type)	All tooth types	Maxillary premolars	Single-rooted teeth/molars with no neighboring teeth	All tooth types	All tooth types
Buccolingual extension of the intraosseous defect	Buccal (for palatal extension)/lingual (for buccal extension)	Buccal/lingual (wide, long beveled palatal incisions recommended)	Lingual	Buccal/lingual	Buccal/lingual

Reasons for selecting the SFA

The elevation of a single flap to access the intraosseous defect allows for several clinical advantages:

* By leaving a great volume of supracrestal soft tissues intact, the vascular supply may reestablish more quickly.
* The SFA may facilitate flap repositioning and suturing; the flap can be easily stabilized to the undetached papilla, thus optimizing wound closure for primary intention healing.
* Wound stabilization and preservation of an intact interdental papilla may contribute to enhanced preservation of the preexisting gingival esthetics.

As shown in Table 4-1, the SFA is indicated in the presence of varying anatomical conditions known to affect the selection of flap design (see Fig 4-5). Such advantages and flexibility in the indications for this simplified procedure led to several SFA variants, which are all characterized by the elevation of a single, full-thickness buccal flap to access the intraosseous defect.[34–36]

In 2008, Checchi et al[34] modified the original technique of the SFA by coronally advancing the flap with the intention to minimize the esthetic impairment related to the surgical procedure and optimize soft tissue closure at the incision margin. This technique was referred to as the *coronally positioned single-flap approach* (CP-SFA). The modified minimally invasive surgical technique (M-MIST) was proposed in 2009.[35] A substantial overlapping exists between M-MIST and buccal SFA, including aspects related to the interdental flap incision and flap management. However, in the M-MIST, the mesiodistal extension of the incision is kept at minimum (ideally, within the midbuccal area of the involved teeth) to allow for the reflection of a triangular buccal flap. More recently, Zucchelli et al[36] combined the SFA with a connective tissue graft to treat challenging intraosseous defects associated with Miller class IV gingival recessions.

Overall, the results stemming from these SFA variants confirmed the effectiveness of the simplified procedure in improving the clinical conditions of deep vertical lesions while minimizing the invasiveness of the surgical intervention.

Clinical advantages of the SFA

It must be reinforced that adequate surgical access to provide proper root/defect instrumentation of the intraosseous lesion is paramount in the clinical and histologic outcomes. In this respect, the extension and morphology of the defect represents a key aspect when selecting a flap design. On the other hand, data from recent studies indicate that the application of SFA principles may lead to improved clinical outcomes compared with the double-flap approach (DFA)—that is, when anatomical conditions permit.

Therefore, a recent study evaluated whether and to what extent the clinical outcomes of a surgical root debridement are similar when performed by either a SFA or a DFA (according to modified/simplified papilla preservation techniques).[37] All the defects were two- or three-walled intraosseous defects, and no regenerative devices were used in addition to the surgical access (Fig 4-17). At 6 months, treatment with the SFA resulted in significantly greater CAL gain (4.5 mm vs 3.4 mm) and probing depth (PD) reduction (5.2 mm vs 3.9 mm) compared with the DFA[37] (Fig 4-18a). In contrast, postsurgery recession increase was similarly low in both treatment groups (0.7 mm for SFA and 0.5 mm for DFA). Similarly, when deep intraosseous defects received surgical debridement with the additional use of a regenerative agent (recombinant human platelet-derived growth factor BB [rhPDGF-BB] in a β-tricalcium phosphate [β-TCP] carrier), a trend toward a greater CAL gain and PD reduction was observed in the SFA group than the DFA group (Fig 4-18b).

In light of these findings, it appears that the surgical access according to the SFA principles seems to optimize the clinical outcomes following the treatment of deep intraosseous defects when compared with double-flap papilla preservation procedures. Clinical advantages for SFA are evident whether or not a regenerative device is used.

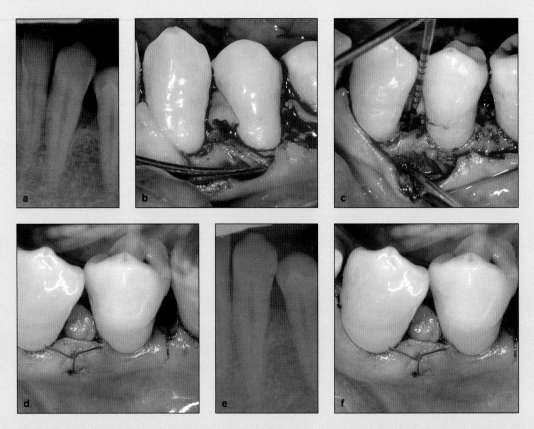

Fig 4-17 Treatment of an intraosseous defect with the SFA without regenerative devices. *(a)* Radiographic view of the lesion at the distal aspect of a mandibular left canine. *(b)* The defect was accessed by a buccal SFA. The interproximal papilla was left intact. *(c)* The defect was mainly three-walled with an intraosseous component of 4 mm. *(d)* At the completion of the surgical debridement, the defect was left to fill with a blood clot, and primary intention healing was obtained by two internal mattress sutures. *(e and f)* Radiograph and clinical view of the defect 6 months after treatment.

Early wound stability following the SFA

Primary intention healing has been recognized as a significant determinant of periodontal wound healing following regenerative procedures.[38–40] In particular, the first postoperative weeks seem to be critical for the maintenance of wound stability.[40–42] Early wound dehiscence may compromise wound stability, which in turn would jeopardize the biologic events leading to periodontal regeneration.[43]

Data from several studies on the early postoperative healing following the elevation of a single mucoperiosteal flap either alone or in combination with regenerative devices results in a high proportion of sites showing complete flap closure during the first postoperative weeks[34,43–46] (Figs 4-19a and 4-19b).[47] In particular, a retrospective analysis of defects treated

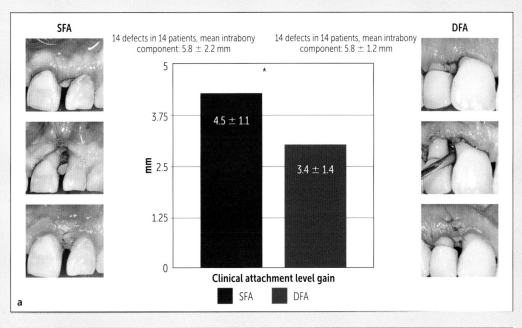

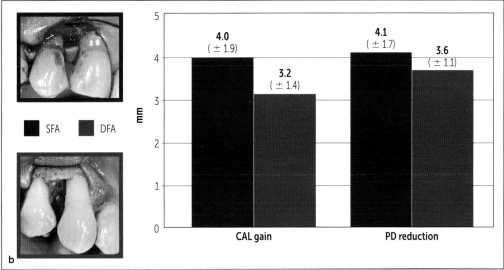

Fig 4-18 *(a)* Six-month CAL gain after treatment of deep, two- to thee-wall intraosseous defects with either the SFA or DFA. No regenerative devices were used. Results showed a significantly greater CAL gain in SFA group (4.5 mm) than DFA group (3.4 mm) at 6 months following surgery.[37] *(b)* Six-month CAL gain and PD reduction after treatment of deep intraosseous defects with SFA or DFA in association with rhPDGF-BB plus β-TCP (GEM 21S, Lynch Biologics [formerly Osteohealth]).[46]

with SFA[45] consistently showed that 84% of defects showed a complete closure of the incision wounds at 2 weeks, as assessed by the early healing index (EHI).[47] In addition, 54% of the treated defects showed optimal conditions of wound closure (ie, EHI = 1). The results also suggest an impact of the different early healing patterns on the 6-month clinical outcomes of the procedure,[45] with a trend toward better clinical outcomes (ie, greater CAL gain, less buccal recession increase) when defects showed optimal wound closure compared with incomplete wound closure (Fig 4-19c).

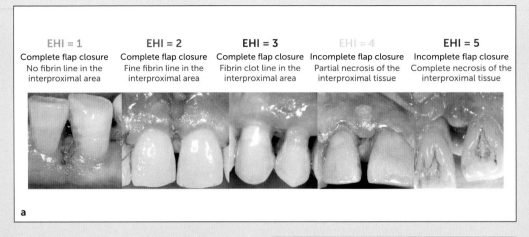

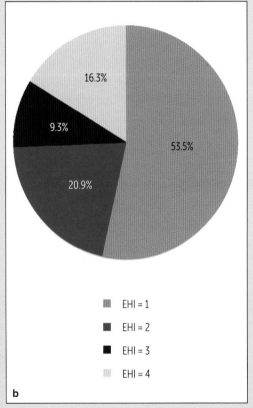

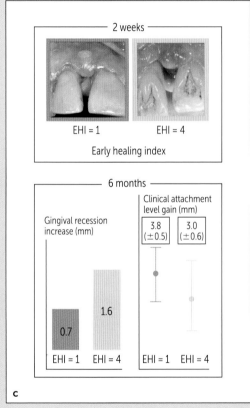

Fig 4-19 *(a)* Early wound healing of the incision at the level of the interdental papilla can be evaluated with the use of a visual index called the early healing index (EHI) as described by Wachtel et al.[47] EHI evaluates the condition of the wound margin using a five-point scale: (1) complete flap closure, no fibrin line in the interproximal area (EHI = 1); (2) complete flap closure, fine fibrin line in the interproximal area (EHI = 2); (3) complete flap closure, fibrin clot in the interproximal area (EHI = 3); (4) incomplete flap closure, partial necrosis of the interproximal tissue (EHI = 4); and (5) incomplete flap closure, complete necrosis of the interproximal tissue (EHI = 5). Scores 1 to 3 are compatible with complete flap closure, whereas the scores 4 and 5 indicate partial or complete tissue necrosis, leading to incomplete flap closure. Score 1 represents optimal wound closure, whereas score 5 refers to the worst healing. *(b)* Farina et al[45] evaluated the early postoperative healing following buccal SFA in the treatment of deep intraosseous periodontal defects. Of the sites with overlying deep intraosseous defects, 36 of 43 (83.7%) showed complete flap closure at 2 weeks, with 53.5% of sites presenting optimal wound closure (EHI = 1) and no sites presenting EHI = 5. *(c)* Comparison of early wound healing and reconstructive outcome between EHI = 1 and EHI = 4.

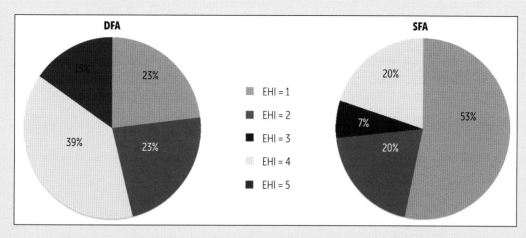

Fig 4-20 Distribution of defects treated with either SFA or DFA in combination with rhPDGF-BB plus β-TCP (GEM 21S) according to EHI, as assessed at 2 weeks following surgery.[46,47]

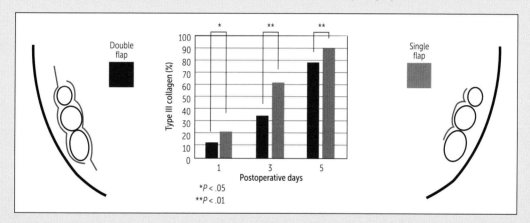

Fig 4-21 Comparison in wound healing dynamics between experimental side (where a single flap was elevated) and control side (where a double flap was elevated). The *red line* shows the incision lines at experimental and control areas. On postoperative days 1, 3, and 5, the proportion of type III collagen–positive area in the defect on the experimental side was greater than the control side.

More recently, a randomized clinical trial demonstrated that SFA may optimize the quality of early wound healing of defects compared with a double-flap papilla preservation technique.[46] At 2 weeks, 12 sites in the SFA group and 6 sites in the DFA group showed complete flap closure (ie, EHI of 1, 2, or 3). The frequency of sites showing optimal wound healing (ie, EHI = 1) was 8 and 3 in the SFA and DFA groups, respectively (Fig 4-20).[46,47] Improved clinical outcomes in the SFA group compared with the DFA group were partly ascribed to enhanced early wound healing.[46]

A recent preclinical study presented a possible explanation for these consistent clinical observations on enhanced early wound healing with the SFA. The effect of a simplified surgical approach was evaluated by comparing the inflammatory cell infiltrate and deposition of type III collagen at days 1, 3, and 5 after periodontal surgery performed with either a limited single flap (experimental site) or a wide double flap (control site).[48] Compared with wide double flaps, the elevation of a limited single flap was associated with a smaller area of the inflammatory infiltrate and a lower amount of neutrophils at day 1 after surgery, faster resolution of postsurgery inflammatory response, more rapid colonization of the elevated gingival tissues by fibroblasts, and greater connective tissue area occupied by type III collagen (Fig 4-21).

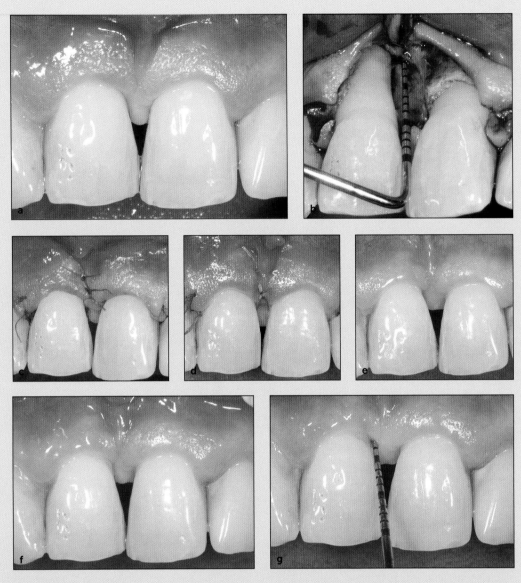

Fig 4-22 The elevation of a single flap to access a periodontal intraosseous defect seems to promote early wound stability, leading to optimal tissue maturation and periodontal regeneration. *(a and b)* Preoperative clinical situation and intrasurgical view of the defect. *(c)* Primary closure at the completion of the surgical procedure. *(d)* Early wound stability: 2 weeks. *(e and f)* Tissue maturation: 3 months and 6 months. *(g)* Long-term stability: 5 years.

Collectively, preclinical and clinical findings seem to support the use of the SFA to access an intraosseous defect to optimize early wound healing (Fig 4-22).

Postsurgery morbidity following the SFA vs the DFA

A historical comparison[1] highlighted differences in surgical time and postsurgery pain when different flap designs are used for regenerative procedures. Surgical chair time was the longest when large papilla preservation flaps and membranes were applied, shorter when large papilla

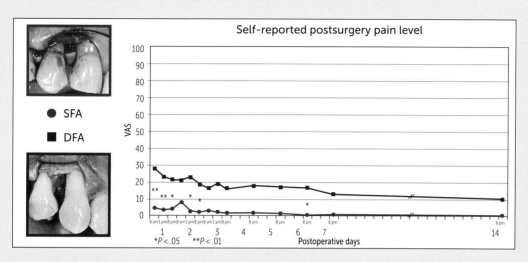

Fig 4-23 The SFA results in lower pain during the first postoperative days than the DFA (VAS scale 0 to 100 mm).

preservation flaps were combined with amelogenins, and by far the shortest when the minimally invasive surgical technique and amelogenins were used.[14,49,50] The number of patients reporting postoperative pain was similar in the two papilla preservation flap studies and much reduced in the minimally invasive surgical technique study, as were pain intensity and consumption of painkillers. From this indirect evidence, the authors concluded that postoperative pain is apparently not influenced by the type of regenerative material but by the type of surgical approach. Visual analog scale (VAS) scores (on a scale of 0 to 100 mm) ranged from an average of 28 mm for an SPPT/MPPT to 19 mm for a minimally invasive procedure.

Patients treated with the SFA reported significantly lower pain levels during the first postoperative days compared with patients undergoing a DFA with SPPT/MPPT.[46] The mean number of analgesics consumed during the first 2 postoperative weeks was 2.73 in the SFA group and 8.69 in the DFA group, with a significantly greater dose of analgesics being used in the DFA group than the SFA group (3.2 versus 1.1, respectively) at day 1 (Fig 4-23). These results were supported by data from clinical trials on M-MIST that consistently showed low postoperative pain levels and a limited consumption of analgesics.[35,44] In the study by Cortellini and Tonetti,[44] none of the patients experienced postoperative pain during the first week following single-flap surgery. Average VAS scores for postoperative discomfort ranged from 10.7 to 12.3. Similarly, low pain levels were reported by Aimetti et al[51] following treatment of deep intraosseous defects treated with the SFA in combination with enamel matrix derivative (EMD). The VAS score in the SFA group was similar to those recorded in the nonsurgical periodontal treatment group (Fig 4-24).

Overall, the available data support a lower postsurgery morbidity following SFA when compared with DFA; the levels of postsurgery pain are in the range of those experienced following a nonsurgical treatment.

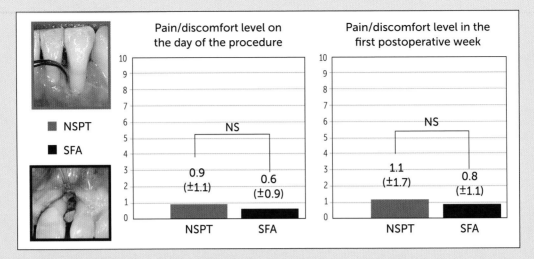

Fig 4-24 When compared with nonsurgical periodontal treatment (NSPT), the SFA results in a similarly low level of pain and discomfort both on the day of the procedure and after the first postoperative week (VAS scale 0 to 10 cm).[51] NS, not significant.

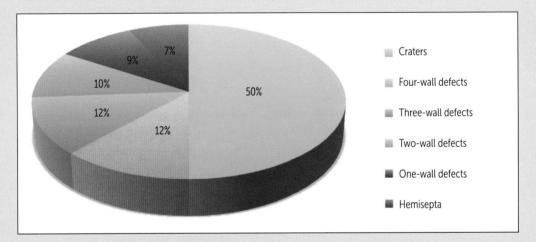

Fig 4-25 Distribution of intraosseous defects according to bone morphology.[52]

How frequently to use the SFA

Obviously, a mandatory prerequisite to apply SFA principles is that the morphology of the defect is compatible with a thorough root/defect debridement when accessed by either the buccal or lingual/palatal side only. Whenever the buccal or lingual/palatal extension of the defect prevents the successful removal of the dental biofilm from the root surface as well as the complete degranulation of the intraosseous component of the defect, conventional DFAs should be performed. However, epidemiologic considerations[52,53] on the morphology of the intraosseous defects seem to suggest that a single surgical access may be possible in a substantial proportion of vertical osseous defects.

The largest epidemiologic study performed on 981 periodontal intraosseous defects[52] described the distribution of the lesions according to bone morphology. Craters represented

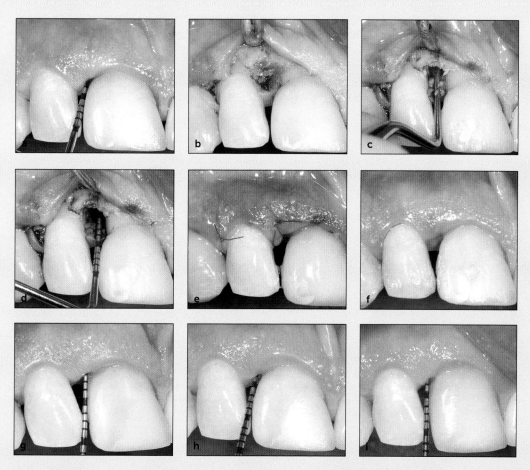

Fig 4-26 *(a)* Persistent bleeding 8-mm pocket at the distal aspect of a right maxillary central incisor. *(b)* Elevation of a buccal mucoperiosteal single flap. *(c)* Surgical debridement with manual instruments. *(d)* The defect was mainly three-walled with a 5-mm-deep intraosseous component. *(e)* Primary intention closure. *(f)* Complete wound closure (EHI = 1) at 2 weeks.[47] *(g)* Clinical view 6 months after surgery. *(h)* Clinical view 1 year after surgery. *(i)* Clinical view 3 years after surgery.

the highest prevalence of defects, followed by four- and three-wall defects and then two-wall defects. One-wall defects and hemisepta accounted for the lowest proportion (Fig 4-25).[52] Moreover, a retrospective trial on 100 dry mandibles[53] showed that the great majority of the craters had a lingual cortical plate at a more coronal level than the buccal cortical plate.

If the morphology of the defect (in terms of residual bone walls) is matched to proper surgical access (either single or double flap), it becomes evident that only a four-wall (circumferential) defect or an interproximal lesion with both buccal and lingual/palatal extension necessarily calls for a DFA. Thus, the SFA (mostly performed on the buccal aspect) seems to represent a suitable surgical access in a relevant proportion of intraosseous defects with different morphologic characteristics (Fig 4-26).[47]

SURGICAL PROTOCOL FOR THE SFA

Presurgical protocol

It should be borne in mind that the SFA is part of the periodontal treatment planning for an intraosseous defect. Therefore, as an option of the corrective treatment phase, the SFA must always be preceded by the cause-related therapy that includes instruction and motivating the patient to achieve a high level of self-performed plaque control as well as full-mouth supra- and subgingival professional mechanical plaque removal (see chapter 3). The surgical procedure should be performed when excellent tissue tone and minimal inflammation of the supracrestal soft tissue is reached following nonsurgical instrumentation. Edematous, inflamed tissues are difficult to manipulate and suture, and postsurgical shrinkage is uncontrolled.

Assessing whether a defect can be accessed with the SFA

To plan the appropriate flap design and regenerative technology, it is paramount to have an accurate diagnosis and identification of the extension and morphology of the defect. Probing to bone under local anesthesia (ie, bone sounding) has been shown to be a valid method to identify the alveolar bone margin (when combined with a periapical radiograph) as a closed procedure[54,55] (Videos 4-2 and 4-3).

Data showed high accuracy of CBCT in detecting intrabony defect morphology compared with periapical radiographs.[56,57] Particularly in maxillary molars, CBCT was useful for detecting furcation involvement and morphology of surrounding periodontal tissues. However, the higher radiation doses and cost-benefit ratio should be carefully considered before using CBCT for diagnosis and treatment planning for intraosseous defects.[58] Therefore, presurgery bone sounding matched with a periapical radiograph performed with the paralleling technique are key to detect the presence, morphology (buccolingual/palatal extension), and depth of the intrabony component of the defect.

Creating the incision line

As previously discussed, the basic principle behind the SFA is the elevation of a full-thickness envelope flap without vertical releasing incisions (Video 4-4). Thus, the incision line is of utmost importance to define the surgical access in term of both flap extension and tissue preservation.

In the event of extensive defects as diagnosed by bone sounding, sulcular incisions are performed on the buccal or lingual/palatal aspect at the teeth adjacent to the defect. At the level of the interdental papilla overlying the intraosseous defect, a horizontal or slightly oblique butt-joint incision is made to maintain the bulk of the interproximal supracrestal soft tissues without thinning the area of the incision line (Fig 4-27). To ensure proper flap elevation without tension, an internally beveled incision may be prolonged to involve the adjacent papillae. The mesiodistal extension of the flap is kept as limited as possible while ensuring proper access for defect debridement and positioning/application of a regenerative device (see Fig 4-27). No attempt is made to remove the supracrestal granulation tissue (if present).

The distance between the tip of the papilla and the horizontal interdental incision is based on the apicocoronal dimension of the supracrestal soft tissues. Presurgical bone sounding must be carefully performed to properly assess the horizontal bone loss and therefore the apicocoronal dimension of the soft tissues overlying the bone crest. The greater the distance from the tip of the papilla to the bone crest (as assessed on the tooth adjacent to the defect), the more apical (ie, close to the base of the papilla) the incision in the interdental area. On the other hand, the incision line must be placed at least 2 mm coronal to the bone crest to ensure adequate access to the intrabony component of the defect for debridement and graft positioning (Fig 4-28).[59] Therefore, the incision line should accomplish both of the following objectives:

- Provide the largest amount of untouched supracrestal soft tissue connected to the undetached papilla to ensure flap revascularization through adaptation and suturing
- Warrant proper access to the intraosseous defect for debridement and, when needed, positioning of the regenerative device

The following guidelines are recommended for specific anatomical situations:

- In case of a wide interproximal space or in the presence of a diastema with a substantial amount of horizontal component of the defect, the incision line may be kept more apical, retaining all the papillary thickness (Video 4-5).
- In case of a narrow interproximal space with a coronal position of the bone crest, the butt-joint incision line needs be kept more coronal (Video 4-6).
- In case of a flat papilla (Video 4-7) or in the presence of a high frenum insertion (Video 4-8), the incision of the papilla overlying the defect can be beveled (instead of being butt-joint) to increase the area of contact between flap and papilla at suturing.
- Incisions are usually performed with a 15C blade; in case of narrow interproximal space or thin biotypes, the use of a microblade may be recommended (Fig 4-29).[60]

How to elevate the flap

The defect is approached by elevating a flap only on the buccal or lingual/palatal aspect (Fig 4-30) and leaving the opposite portion of the interdental supracrestal soft tissues undetached. The full-thickness elevation of the marginal portion of the flap is performed with the use of a microsurgical periosteal elevator (Fig 4-31).[61] Flap reflection should be minimized to limit the vascular damage caused by flap elevation.[62–65] Although unnecessary separation of the gingiva from the underlying bone should be avoided, proper access to root and defect by a tension-free flap is mandatory.

Incision line

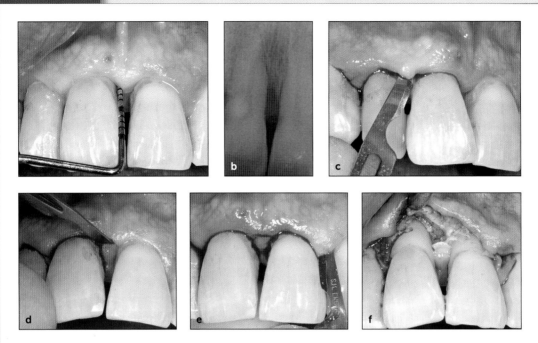

Fig 4-27 *(a)* Preoperative defect located at the mesial aspect of a maxillary central incisor. *(b)* Radiographic view. *(c)* An internal beveled incision was performed at the interdental papilla mesial to the defect. *(d)* At the level of the interdental papilla overlying the intraosseous defect, a horizontal butt-joint incision was made. The palatal portion of the interdental supracrestal soft tissues was left undetached. *(e)* The flap was extended distally with an internal bevel incision. *(f)* Flap elevation provides full access to the osseous lesion and root surface.

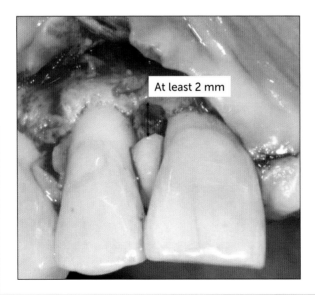

At least 2 mm

Fig 4-28 The incision line must be placed at least 2 mm coronal to the bone crest. This will ensure adequate access to the intrabony component of the defect for defect debridement and graft positioning and provide an adequate amount of supracrestal soft tissue to guarantee the vascular supply of the interdental papilla and adaptation of the sutures. (Reprinted with permission from Farina et al.[59])

Buccal SFA in the presence of a narrow papilla

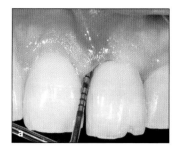 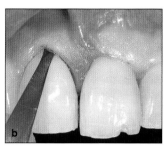 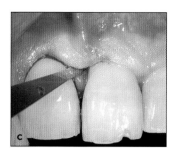

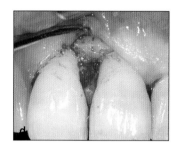

Fig 4-29 *(a)* Preoperative bone sounding at the defect located at the mesial aspect of a maxillary central incisor. *(b and c)* A microblade was used for the intrasulcular incision as well as for the incision at the base of the interproximal papilla. *(d)* A limited single buccal flap was elevated. (Reprinted with permission from Trombelli et al.[60])

SFA with a palatal approach

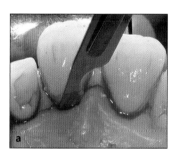 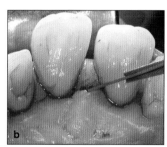 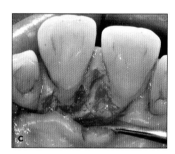

Fig 4-30 Following an intrasulcular *(a)* and butt-joint incision *(b)*, a full-thickness flap was elevated *(c)* on the palatal aspect, leaving the buccal portion of the interdental supracrestal soft tissues undetached.

Flap elevation

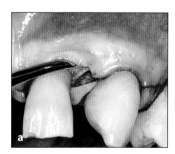 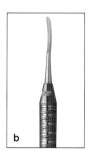

Fig 4-31 *(a and b)* Flap reflection is performed by using a microsurgical periosteal elevator (P-TROM periosteal elevator, Hu-Friedy). (Reprinted with permission from Trombelli et al.[61])

Root and defect debridement

Root and defect debridement is performed using both ultrasonic and hand instruments (Videos 4-9 and 4-10). Hirschfeld file scalers (Hu-Friedy) are particularly indicated to remove granulation tissues and decorticalize the bony walls of the defect. Root debridement is performed with mechanical ultrasonic instrumentation. If there are anomalies or irregularities, fine diamond burs and mini five Langer curettes (Hu-Friedy) may be used to create a more regular root morphology (Video 4-11). Cortical perforations can be performed in the presence of corticalized bone walls, which has been shown to improve the clinical outcomes in spontaneously healed intraosseous defects[66] (Video 4-12).

Suturing technique

Usually, wound closure is obtained by two internal mattress sutures (Figs 4-32 and Fig 4-33, Video 4-13). A first horizontal internal mattress suture is placed coronal to the mucogingival junction between the flap and the base of the opposite (either lingual/palatal or buccal) intact papilla to relocate the flap to its original position. Then, a second horizontal internal mattress suture is placed between the most coronal portion of the flap (in proximity to the incision line) and the most coronal portion of the papilla to ensure primary closure.

When needed (eg, in case of a large, thick interdental papilla), multiple internal mattress sutures (Video 4-14) or additional interrupted sutures (Video 4-15) may be performed to improve conditions for primary intention healing at the incision line. Sutures should not exert excessive tension on the flap (passive adaptation).

In case of narrow interproximal space, a modified internal mattress suture may be preferred to limit tissue trauma from suturing (Video 4-16). The remaining interdental papillae included in the surgical area are passively repositioned by simple interrupted sutures or modified internal mattress sutures (Fig 4-34). 6-0 Vicryl sutures (Johnson & Johnson) are commonly used and left in place for at least 14 days. This will ensure flap closure until sufficient wound maturation is reached to resist disruptive mechanical forces acting on the wound margins.

Accessing multiple defects with the SFA

The SFA can be effectively used to treat multiple intraosseous defects in the same surgical area, provided the morphology and extension of the lesions can ensure proper surgical access by elevating a single (buccal or lingual/palatal) flap. Surgical steps, including incision line, flap elevation, and suturing technique, will reflect those described for the treatment of a single defect (Fig 4-35).

Suturing technique

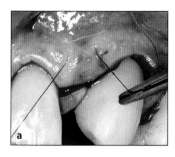
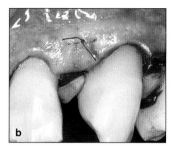
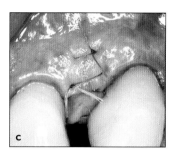

Fig 4-32 *(a and b)* A first horizontal internal mattress suture was placed between the buccal flap and the base of the attached lingual papilla coronal to the mucogingival junction to reposition the buccal flap. *(c)* A second internal mattress suture was placed between the most coronal portion of the flap and the most coronal portion of the palatal papilla to ensure wound closure by primary intention.

Suture of a palatal flap

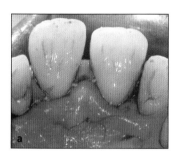
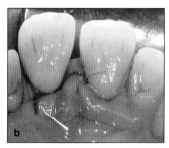
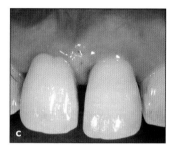

Fig 4-33 Suture of a palatal SFA. *(a)* A first horizontal internal mattress suture was placed between the palatal flap and the base of the attached buccal papilla to reposition the palatal flap. *(b)* A second internal mattress suture was placed close to the incision line for primary closure. *(c)* Buccal aspect following suture.

Suturing technique at interdental papillae adjacent to the defect

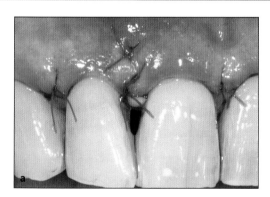
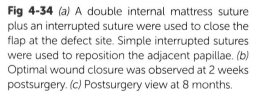
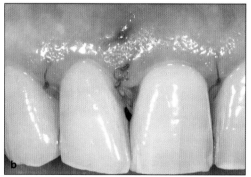
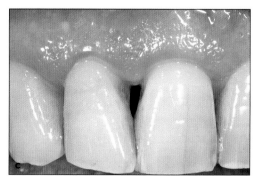

Fig 4-34 *(a)* A double internal mattress suture plus an interrupted suture were used to close the flap at the defect site. Simple interrupted sutures were used to reposition the adjacent papillae. *(b)* Optimal wound closure was observed at 2 weeks postsurgery. *(c)* Postsurgery view at 8 months.

Treatment of multiple intraosseous defects

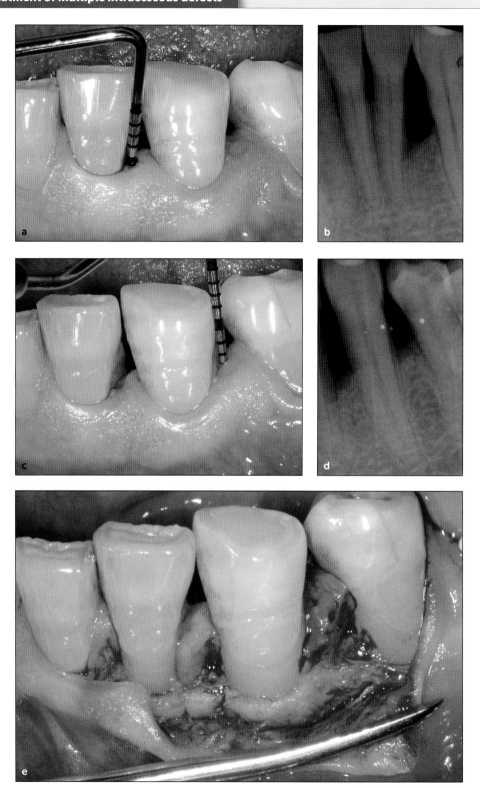

Fig 4-35 Surgical debridement of two contiguous intraosseous defects accessed with the SFA. *(a and b)* Preoperative CAL loss at the distal aspect of a mandibular left lateral incisor. *(c and d)* Preoperative CAL loss at the distal aspect of a mandibular left canine. *(e)* The extension of the flap was kept limited while ensuring proper access to the defects.

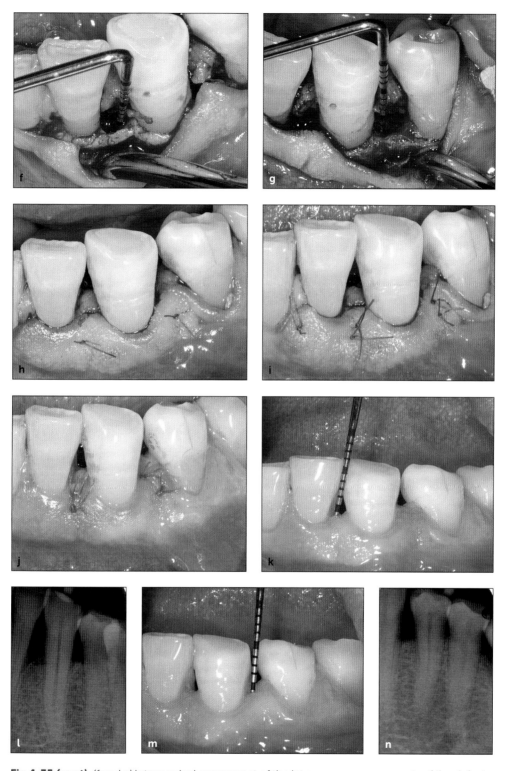

Fig 4-35 (cont) *(f and g)* Intrasurgical assessment of the intraosseous components of the defects. *(h and i)* A horizontal internal mattress suture at the base of the papillae and a second internal mattress suture at the most coronal portion of the papillae. *(j)* Clinical view at suture removal (2 weeks postsurgery). *(k to n)* Clinical and radiographic assessment of lateral incisor *(k and l)* and canine *(m and n)* 2 years after surgery.

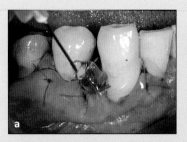
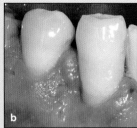

Fig 4-36 *(a)* At the completion of the suture, a local agent (Aminogam, Professional Dietetics) was positioned at the incision area to facilitate early healing. *(b)* Complete wound closure and absence of fibrin line in the interproximal area (EHI = 1) were observed 2 weeks postsurgery.

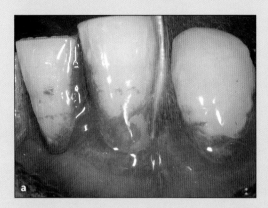
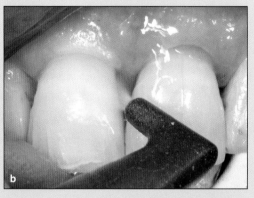

Fig 4-37 During the recall session, the supra- and juxtagingival dental biofilm is thoroughly removed at regenerated sites with ultrasonic instruments *(a)* or airflow *(b)*.

Postsurgery regimen

Following the SFA regenerative procedure, the following actions are indicated:

- Avoid any surgical dressings. Surgical dressings may create undesirable compression of the surgical flap and allow excessive plaque accumulation on the healing site.
- Ensure the patient refrains from mechanical oral hygiene procedures in the area for at least 4 to 6 weeks. Early mechanical disturbance of the healing site may be detrimental for the reconstructive outcome. The patient should use 0.12% chlorhexidine mouthrinse (two to three times daily) with antidiscoloration system, along with weekly professional removal of supra- and juxtagingival plaque (Fig 4-36). Systemic antibiotics may be prescribed; however, there is no evidence that a postsurgical antibiotic regimen has a positive effect on the regenerative outcome.[67] Local agents that may facilitate early healing (Fig 4-37) may be recommended for professional and patient use during the first 2 weeks after surgery.
- Ensure the patient refrains from smoking or limits their daily cigarette consumption. Smoking has been consistently associated with impaired healing response following reconstructive procedures.[8,68] A trend toward an impaired treatment outcome has recently been shown in heavy compared with light smokers following SFA combined with graft biomaterial and EMD[9] (Fig 4-38).
- Enroll the patient in a supportive therapy program at monthly intervals for the first 3 months and every 3 months thereafter.
- Avoid probing or deep subgingival instrumentation at the treated site for at least 6 months postsurgery.

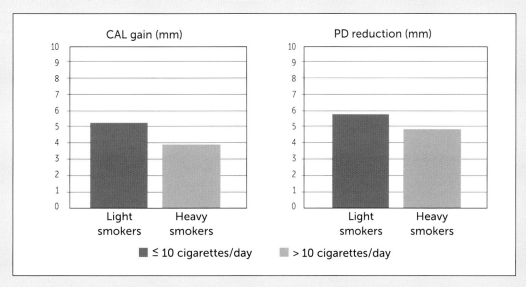

Fig 4-38 Patients smoking more than 10 cigarettes per day showed a tendency to a lower CAL gain and PD reduction compared with patients smoking up to 10 cigarettes per day.

REGENERATIVE DEVICES WITH THE SFA

Necessity of regenerative devices

The surgical access based on the elevation of a single flap represents a valuable treatment even when used as a standalone protocol (ie, without the additional use of reconstructive devices or bioactive agents)[33,37,44,69] (Fig 4-39). According to recent studies, the magnitude of CAL gain observed for single-flap procedures without the use of reconstructive devices (ranging on average from 2.6 to 4.5 mm) can be compared with the outcomes achieved with double-flap procedures in association with membranes[4,8,30] or EMD.[67,70,71]

Overall, these observations highlight the great potential of the SFA procedure to allow for a faster revascularization of the surgical area, which may facilitate healing by primary intention, and greater wound stability postsurgery, allowing for uneventful tissue formation and maturation. The undetached papilla prevents the collapse of the soft tissues, maintaining space for regeneration.

The potential of the SFA procedures to treat intraosseous lesions may partly explain the findings from three randomized controlled trials evaluating the additional use of a regenerative technology.[33,44,69] In essence, the results from these studies failed to find any significant additional benefit from the use of a resorbable membrane with bone substitutes,[33] EMD with or without a xenograft,[44] or rhPDGF-BB[69] when combined with a simplified single-flap procedure. Blood clot protection is warranted by the residual bony walls, the root surface, the buccal or lingual/palatal soft tissues, and the "lid" of the intact interdental papilla (Fig 4-40). These findings seem to suggest that the influence of the flap design on

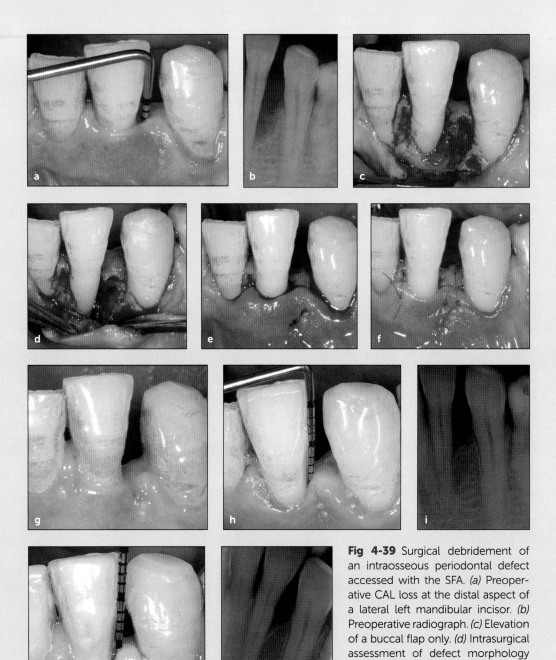

Fig 4-39 Surgical debridement of an intraosseous periodontal defect accessed with the SFA. *(a)* Preoperative CAL loss at the distal aspect of a lateral left mandibular incisor. *(b)* Preoperative radiograph. *(c)* Elevation of a buccal flap only. *(d)* Intrasurgical assessment of defect morphology and severity. The root was thoroughly debrided and the defect left to fill with a blood clot. *(e and f)* The flap was closed for healing by primary intention. *(g)* Suture removal 2 weeks after surgery. *(h and i)* Probing and radiograph after 12 months. *(j and k)* Probing and radiograph after 8 years. (Reprinted with permission from Trombelli et al.[37])

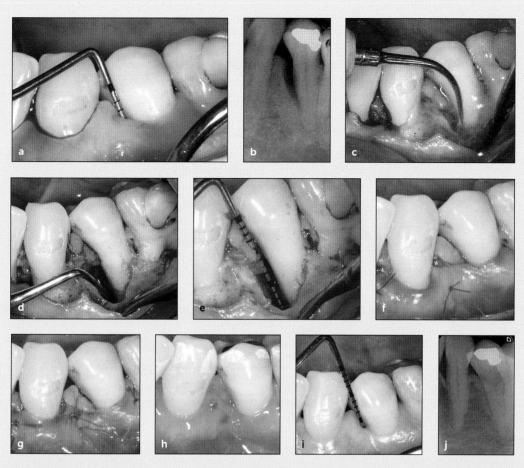

Fig 4-40 Treatment of a periodontal intraosseous defect with the SFA without regenerative devices. *(a)* Preoperative CAL loss at the mesiobuccal aspect of a left mandibular first premolar. *(b)* Preoperative radiograph. *(c and d)* The elevation of a buccal mucoperiosteal flap allowed for proper root/defect debridement. *(e)* The defect was characterized by a narrow angle and a 7-mm-deep one- to two-wall intraosseous component. The defect was left filled with blood clot only. *(f and g)* Suturing technique. *(h)* Complete wound closure (EHI = 1) at 2 weeks after surgery. *(i and j)* Clinical and radiographic views at 9 years after treatment.

clinical outcomes may exceed that of the regenerative technology.[72] However, the findings regarding the high predictability of the single-flap procedure must be interpreted in view of the following aspects:

- *Baseline defect characteristics.* In these studies,[33,44,69] defect selection resulted in mainly two- to three-walled defects with a narrow defect angle, which are characterized by enhanced healing response.[49,73] Therefore, it is possible to speculate that the added value of a single-flap procedure becomes more evident especially in defects prone to spontaneous healing.

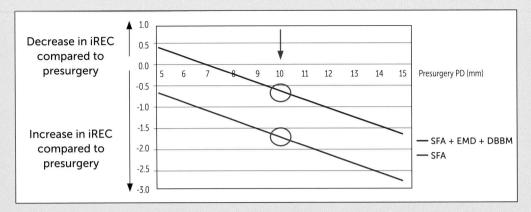

Fig 4-41 On the basis of the bivariate model proposed by Farina et al,[75] a presurgery PD of 10 mm may result in 1.7 mm interproximal gingival recession (iREC) in defects treated with SFA alone or 0.7 mm in defects treated with SFA in combination with EMD and DBBM.

- *Histologic considerations.* Healing after raising an access flap is expected to be histologically different from a regenerative surgery. Periodontal regeneration can be obtained after the use of a variety of bone grafts and substitutes, GTR, biologic factors, and combinations (see chapter 2). On the contrary, healing after raising an access flap is predominantly characterized by repair (ie, formation of a long junctional epithelium) and no or limited regeneration. Differences in histologic healing (regeneration vs repair) may be considered as a potential factor affecting the long-term stability of the clinical results.[74]
- *Postoperative gingival recession.* The recession of the gingival margin following the SFA was generally within 1 mm (range: 0.1 to 1.5 mm) at 6 to 12 months postoperatively. Although these simplified approaches may minimize the surgical trauma during the manipulation of soft tissues, a high heterogeneity in recession change was observed among and within studies. A retrospective analysis was conducted to evaluate the influence of patient-related and site-specific factors as well as the adopted reconstructive strategy on recession change at 6 months after the treatment of intraosseous defects with the SFA.[75] The results of the study showed that interproximal recession increase is significantly limited by the regenerative technology. In particular, defects treated with open flap debridement alone are more prone to show an increase in interproximal gingival recession than defects treated with graft material in combination with bioactive agents (ie, deproteinized bovine bone mineral [DBBM] + EMD; Fig 4-41).[75]

Which regenerative device to use

Guided tissue regeneration

The use of GTR as an efficacious regenerative procedure in the treatment of intraosseous periodontal defects has been widely validated both histologically[76–79] (see chapter 2) and clinically.[79]

GTR with a resorbable membrane has been successfully used to treat deep intraosseous lesions in association with the SFA. A randomized controlled trial[33] was performed to evaluate the adjunctive effect of GTR with a resorbable membrane and a hydroxyapatite (HA)-based graft in the treatment of periodontal intraosseous defects accessed with the SFA (Figs 4-42 to 4-44).[29,61,80]

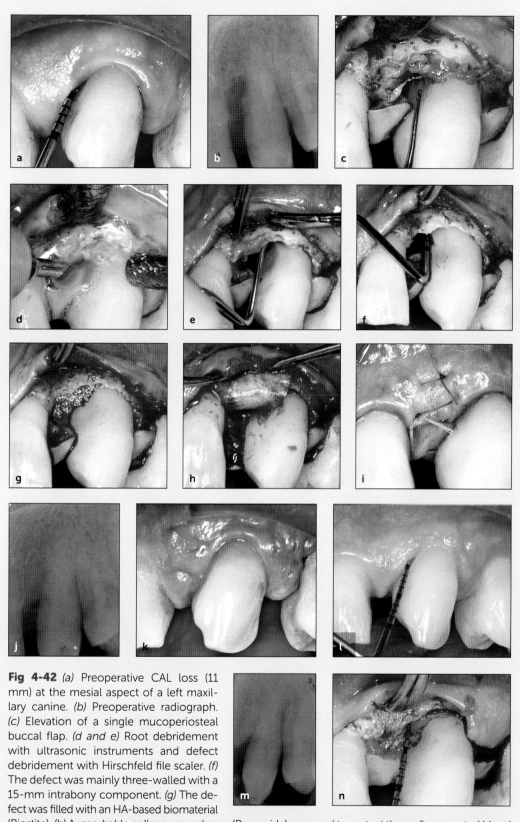

Fig 4-42 *(a)* Preoperative CAL loss (11 mm) at the mesial aspect of a left maxillary canine. *(b)* Preoperative radiograph. *(c)* Elevation of a single mucoperiosteal buccal flap. *(d and e)* Root debridement with ultrasonic instruments and defect debridement with Hirschfeld file scaler. *(f)* The defect was mainly three-walled with a 15-mm intrabony component. *(g)* The defect was filled with an HA-based biomaterial (Biostite). *(h)* A resorbable collagen membrane (Paroguide) was used to protect the graft-supported blood clot. *(i)* Suturing technique. *(j)* Periapical radiograph at completion of the surgical procedure. *(k)* Suture removal at 2 weeks after surgery (EHI = 1). *(l and m)* Clinical and radiographic views 9 years after treatment. *(n)* At reentry, a complete resolution of the intrabony component of the defect was evident. (Reprinted with permission from Trombelli et al.[61])

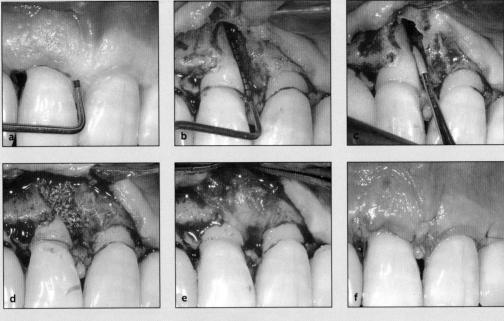

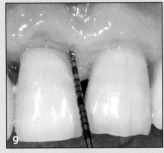

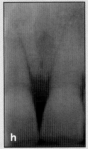

Fig 4-43 Treatment of a periodontal intraosseous defect associated with a cemental tear with SFA and GTR (see Fig 4-2). *(a)* Preoperative view of the surgical site. There was 16 mm of CAL loss evident on the mesial aspect of a central incisor. *(b)* Intrasurgical assessment of the intraosseous component of the defect. The intrabony component was 11 mm deep. *(c)* After debridement, the root surface was smoothened by an ultrafine diamond bur (Intensiv Perio Set, Intensiv). *(d)* The defect was filled with deproteinized bovine bone mineral (Bio-Oss small granules, Geistlich). *(e)* A resorbable collagen membrane (Bio-Gide, Geistlich) was used for GTR provision. *(f)* Wound closure was obtained using internal mattress and interrupted sutures. *(g and h)* Clinical and radiographic views 12 months after treatment. (Reprinted with permission from Simonelli et al.[80])

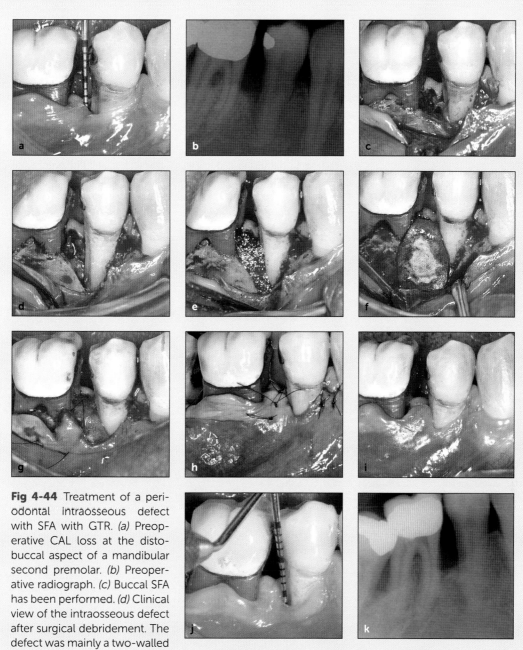

Fig 4-44 Treatment of a periodontal intraosseous defect with SFA with GTR. *(a)* Preoperative CAL loss at the distobuccal aspect of a mandibular second premolar. *(b)* Preoperative radiograph. *(c)* Buccal SFA has been performed. *(d)* Clinical view of the intraosseous defect after surgical debridement. The defect was mainly a two-walled defect. *(e)* The intraosseous component of the defect was grafted with an HA-based biomaterial (Biostite). *(f)* A resorbable collagen membrane (Paroguide) was used for cell occlusion and wound stabilization. *(g and h)* Suturing technique. *(i)* Clinical view at suture removal, 2 weeks after surgery. *(j and k)* Clinical and radiographic views at 8-year follow-up. (Reprinted with permission from Trombelli et al.[29])

Table 4-2 Clinical outcomes of SFA with or without HA graft and GTR in the treatment of peri-odontal intraosseous defects

	CAL gain (mm)	PD reduction (mm)	Recession increase (mm)
SFA	4.4 ± 1.5	5.3 ± 1.5	0.8 ± 0.8
SFA ± HA/GTR	4.7 ± 2.5	5.3 ± 2.4	0.4 ± 1.4

There were 24 intraosseous defects that were randomly allocated to treatment, including the SFA + HA/GTR or the SFA alone. Clinical outcomes assessed at 6 months postsurgery indicated that SFA with and without HA + GTR were similarly effective in the treatment of intraosseous periodontal defects. The SFA + HA/GTR group showed substantial CAL gain (4.7 mm) and PD reduction (5.3 mm) together with limited gingival recession increase (0.4 mm). Similarly, the group treated with the SFA alone showed a CAL gain of 4.4 mm, a PD reduction of 5.3 mm, and a gingival recession increase of 0.8 mm. However, no significant differences between the groups were identified (Table 4-2). This lack of difference between treatments may be partly explained by the optimal conditions for wound healing provided by SFA leading to successful clinical results for the control group as well.

Technically, when a membrane has to be used in conjunction with SFA, the resorbable barrier device has to be trimmed to resemble a pear shape, adapted to defect morphology on either the buccal or lingual aspect, and stabilized by gently elevating the undetached papilla from the overlying defect (Video 4-17). Unfortunately, the use of the membrane barrier may somewhat compromise the revascularization of the surgical site, resulting in early wound dehiscence and thus jeopardizing the final outcome (Fig 4-45). Interestingly, in the authors' study,[33] the SFA + HA/GTR group resulted in incomplete early wound closure in 5 out of 12 defects, whereas the SFA group showed complete wound closure in all defects (Fig 4-46).

In this respect, a consistent decrease in complications was observed when barriers were not incorporated into the surgical procedure. In particular, the adoption of amelogenins largely reduced the prevalence of complications.[81] A randomized controlled trial comparing membranes and EMD showed a relevant difference in complication rate: 100% in the membrane-treated defects, 6% in the EMD-treated sites.[82] These observations leave an open question whether the use of a membrane would represent a suitable regenerative option when matched with the SFA.

Biologic agents

Improved treatment outcomes following the use of bioactive agents with or without bone grafts in association with the SFA have been reported. In particular, the SFA has been investigated in association with two biologic agents:

- rhPDGF-BB
- EMD

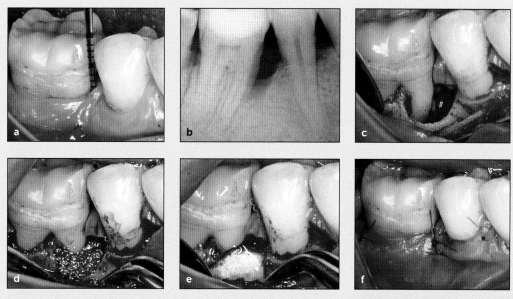

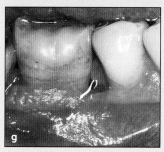

Fig 4-45 SFA with HA graft and GTR in the treatment of a periodontal intraosseous defect at the mesial aspect of a first mandibular molar. *(a and b)* Preoperative CAL loss and radiograph. *(c)* Clinical view of the intraosseous defect after surgical debridement. *(d)* The defect was filled with an HA-based biomaterial. *(e)* The defect was covered with a resorbable collagen membrane, which was stabilized under the papilla. *(f)* Primary intention healing at wound closure. *(g)* Clinical view at suture removal, 2 weeks after surgery. An incomplete flap closure with partial necrosis of the interproximal tissue compatible with an EHI = 4 was evident.

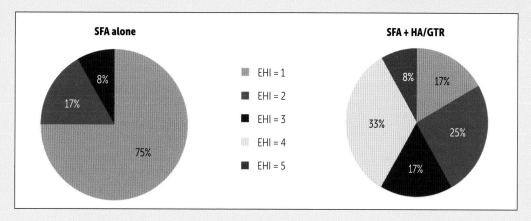

Fig 4-46 Quality of soft tissue healing at 2 weeks after the SFA with or without HA graft and GTR in the treatment of periodontal intraosseous defects (defect distribution according to EHI[47]).

Recombinant human platelet-derived growth factor. According to a systematic review,[83] the use of rhPDGF-BB alone in the treatment of intraosseous defects may result in a significant improvement of clinical outcomes. A significant increase in CAL gain (≤ 1 mm), in linear bone growth (≤ 2 mm), and in percent of bone fill (≤ 40%) compared with controls was reported.

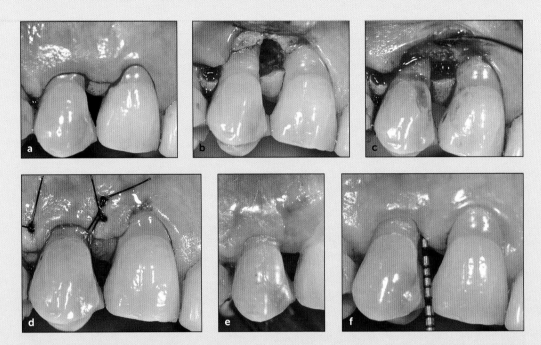

Fig 4-47 Treatment of a periodontal intraosseous defect with a buccal SFA and rhPDGF-BB plus β-TCP (GEM 21S). *(a)* Incision outline. *(b)* A microsurgical periosteal elevator was used to raise a flap only on the buccal aspect. *(c)* The intraosseous component of the defect was treated with rhPDGF-BB in a β-TCP carrier. *(d)* Suturing technique. *(e)* Clinical view at suture removal (2 weeks postsurgery, EHI = 1). *(f)* Probing measurements at 6 months postsurgery. (Reprinted with permission from Schincaglia et al.[46])

A recent randomized clinical trial evaluated the outcomes of a regenerative strategy based on rhPDGF-BB (0.3 mg/mL) and β-TCP in the treatment of intraosseous defects accessed with the SFA versus the DFA. Focusing on 15 defects accessed with the SFA, a significant increase in CAL gain (4.0 ± 1.9 mm) and PD reduction (4.1 ± 1.7 mm) together with a slight (nonsignificant) increase in gingival interproximal recession were observed 6 months after therapy. The improved clinical outcomes in the SFA group may be partially ascribed to the enhanced early wound healing; in fact, at 2 weeks, 12 out of 15 cases showed complete flap closure, with 8 sites showing optimal wound healing (ie, EHI = 1; Fig 4-47).[46]

Enamel matrix derivative. EMD is a biologically active agent capable of promoting periodontal regeneration when applied to a periodontally compromised root surface after surgical debridement (see chapter 2). From a clinical standpoint, the effectiveness of EMD for the treatment of intraosseous defects has been widely reviewed.[84–86] In particular, the meta-analysis proposed by Koop et al[85] showed a statistically significant additional improvement in CAL (1.3 mm) and PD (0.92 mm) in favor of the use of EMD compared with a control (open flap debridement/ethylenediaminetetraacetic acid [EDTA]/placebo) 1 year after therapy.

A series of studies investigated the combination of SFA and EMD[45,59,75] (Figs 4-48 to 4-50; Video 4-18). In the 2014 study by Farina et al,[59] deep periodontal intraosseous defects were treated with a buccal SFA plus EMD. Treatment resulted in a significant CAL gain (3.8 ± 1.0 mm) and PD reduction (4.9 ± 1.8 mm) at 6 months after treatment. A similar CAL gain (4.1 ± 1.2 mm) was reported 12 months after treatment by a randomized controlled trial where an SFA variant (M-MIST technique) was used in association with EMD in intraosseous defects.

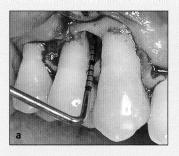
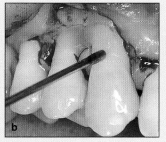
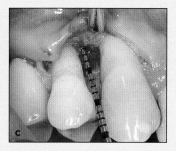

Fig 4-48 *(a)* Intrasurgical view of the deep intraosseous defect at the maxillary right first premolar. *(b)* Following root debridement and conditioning, the defect was treated with EMD. *(c)* Complete resolution of the defect at reentry.

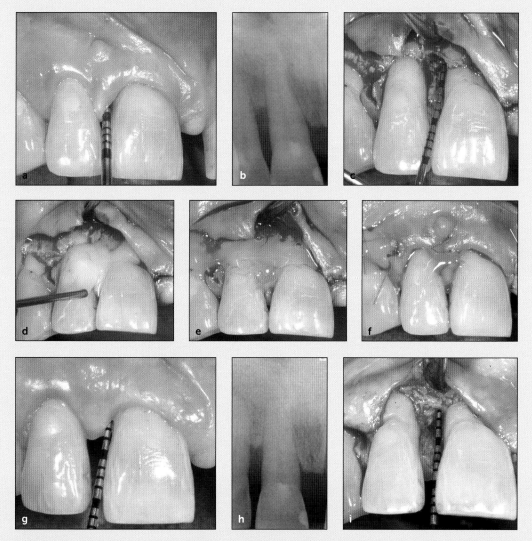

Fig 4-49 *(a and b)* Preoperative probing and radiographic view of an intraosseous defect at the distal aspect of a maxillary central incisor. *(c)* Intrasurgical view following buccal flap elevation. *(d)* The exposed root surface was conditioned with 24% EDTA gel for 2 minutes and then rinsed with saline. *(e)* The EDTA-treated root surface and surrounding bony walls were conditioned with the EMD. *(f)* SFA closed with internal mattress sutures. *(g and h)* Probing measurements and radiographic view at 7 years following surgery. *(i)* Resolution of the defects at reentry. (Parts *a*, *b*, *c*, and *e* reprinted with permission from Farina et al.[59])

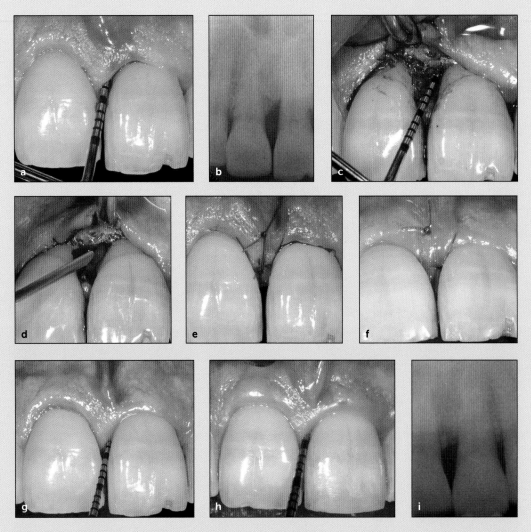

Fig 4-50 *(a)* Persistent bleeding, 8-mm pocket at the mesial aspect of a maxillary central incisor at 6 months following nonsurgical therapy. *(b)* Presurgery radiograph. *(c)* The defect was mainly three-walled with a narrow angle and 6-mm-deep intraosseous component. *(d)* Application of EMD to EDTA-conditioned root surface and defect. *(e)* Flap closure with internal mattress and interrupted sutures. *(f)* Complete wound closure at 2 weeks following surgery. *(g)* Clinical appearance at 1 year following surgery. A CAL gain of 5 mm was achieved. *(h and i)* Probing and radiographic view at 5 years following surgery.

EMD plus additional bone substitute. The use of a bone substitute in combination with EMD in the regenerative treatment of intraosseous defects should also be taken into consideration as a valid regenerative strategy with the following advantages:

- Improvement of the treatment outcomes (CAL gain) in challenging defects with unfavorable morphology (eg, deep intrabony component, wide angle, one- to two-wall morphology)[9,59] (Fig 4-51; Video 4-19)
- Limitation of the postsurgical interproximal gingival recession[45,75,87] (Fig 4-52; Video 4-20)

EMD

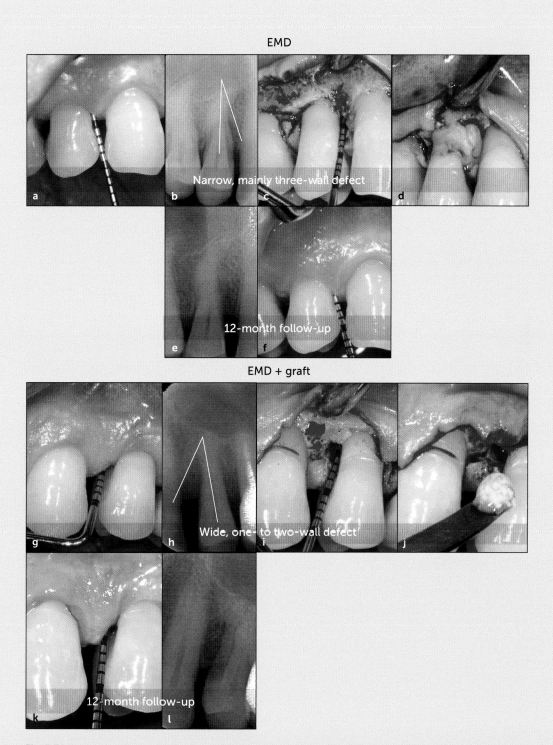

Fig 4-51 EMD with or without graft biomaterials. A mainly three-wall defect with a narrow angle is treated with EMD alone *(a to f)*. A one- to two-wall defect with a wide radiographic angle is treated with a combination of EMD and a graft biomaterial *(g to l)*. (Reprinted with permission from Trombelli et al.[9])

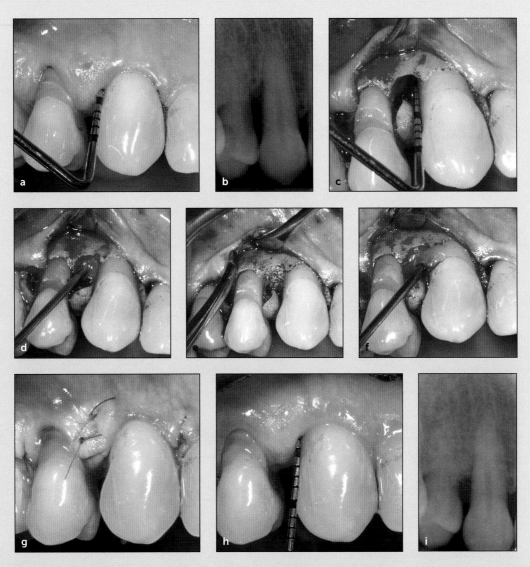

Fig 4-52 *(a)* Preoperative CAL loss at the distal aspect of a maxillary right canine. *(b)* Radiographic view before surgery. *(c)* Intrasurgical view of the intraosseous components of the defect. *(d)* A sandwich technique[87] was applied to stratify EMD and the graft biomaterial (ie, DBBM Bio-Oss small granules). A first layer of EMD was injected to condition the bone defect and the EDTA-treated root surface. *(e)* DBBM mixed with EMD was subsequently positioned to fill the intrabony component of the defect. *(f)* A second layer of EMD was used to cover the grafted DBBM particles and condition the suprabony portion of the root surface as well as supracrestal soft tissues. *(g)* Wound closure after suturing. *(h and i)* Clinical and radiographic views at 12 months after surgery. Note the limited postsurgery recession. (Reprinted with permission from Farina et al.[45])

Because of its gel-like consistency, EMD has a limited spacemaking effect that in turn may potentially affect its regenerative capacity. Therefore, a combined approach using EMD plus a graft biomaterial may be preferred, particularly when the regenerative treatment is directed toward deep intraosseous defects with a noncontained morphology.[88] The rationale for this approach is that, while EMD would exert a biologic effect on the events leading to periodontal regeneration, the use of the graft may somewhat hinder the collapse of the flap into the bone defect and enhance blood clot stability during the early healing phase.

The combination of EMD and a graft biomaterial is applied according to the so-called sandwich technique, as originally proposed by Trombelli et al[87] (Figs 4-53 and 4-54; see Fig 4-52 and Video 4-20):

1. A first layer of EMD is used to condition the bone defect and the most apical portion of the EDTA-treated root surface.
2. Then, graft particles that have been previously mixed with EMD are positioned to graft the intrabony component of the defect up to the bone crest.
3. Finally, the remaining exposed portion of the root surface as well as the supracrestal soft tissues are conditioned by an additional EMD layer.

Several studies investigated the combined effect of EMD plus a graft biomaterial in the treatment of intraosseous defects. A recent meta-analysis reported an adjunctive CAL gain of 0.9 mm when DBBM was combined with EMD.[85] However, the combination of EMD with a biomaterial must be carefully selected considering the morphology of the intraosseous defect, also in view of the additional cost of the combined procedure.[89] In this respect, the prognostic role of defect configuration (in terms of residual bony walls) in EMD-based regenerative periodontal treatment has been well documented. In particular, Tonetti et al[49] found that the probability of reaching a 1-year CAL gain of 3 mm in an EMD-treated intraosseous defect decreased 2.69 times for a one- to two-wall lesion compared with a three-wall lesion.

Although the use of the SFA leads to better conditions for wound stability, the added value of an additional graft to EMD may be seen even when defects with different bone morphology/severity are accessed by a single flap only. In a pragmatic trial, 24 periodontal intraosseous defects were accessed with a buccal SFA and treated with EMD or EMD plus DBBM according to the operator's discretion.[59] Both treatments resulted in substantial CAL gain and PD reduction at 6 months after surgery. However, the morphology of defects treated with EMD and EMD + DBBM was markedly different, with EMD-treated defects showing a dominant three-wall component, while EMD + DBBM defects were predominantly one-wall. When interpreting the results in light of these observations, it appears that deep intraosseous defects with an unfavorable morphology (ie, mainly due to a dominant one-wall component and large defect angle and width) treated with SFA and EMD + DBBM may respond in a similar manner as defects with a more favorable morphology (ie, mainly three-wall component and narrow defect angle and width) treated with SFA + EMD only (see Fig 4-51). A recent study evaluated the cost-effectiveness of different surgical EMD-based procedures for treating intraosseous lesions. The authors conclude that, in cases where EMD application is indicated, the association of EMD with bone grafts (eg, bovine bone substitutes) shows a more advantageous cost-effectiveness ratio than EMD alone.[89]

Recently, the authors introduced a novel, simplified composite outcome measure (COM) to evaluate the clinical effect of different regenerative devices when used in intraosseous defects accessed by SFA.[90] COM is based on the combination of CAL gain (ie, clinical relevance) and postsurgery residual PD (ie, pocket closure). According to COM, treatment is considered as *successful* when a clinically relevant result (ie, a CAL gain ≥ 3 mm) is associated with the

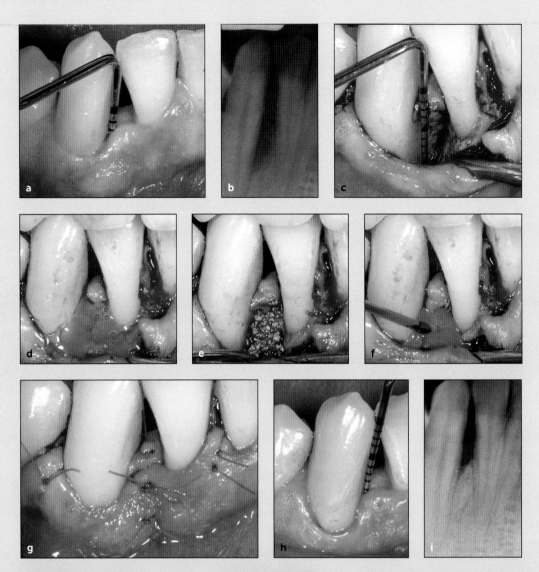

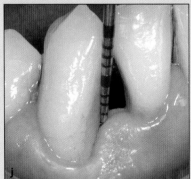

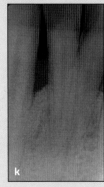

Fig 4-53 *(a)* Preoperative CAL loss at the mesial aspect of a mandibular canine. *(b)* Preoperative radiographic view of the lesion. *(c)* Intrasurgical assessment of the intraosseous characteristics of the defect. The predominantly one- to two- wall defect showed a 9-mm intrabony component. *(d)* A first layer of EMD was injected to condition the bone defect and the EDTA-treated root surface. *(e)* DBBM mixed with EMD to graft the defect up to the bone crest. *(f)* DBBM particles (Bio-Oss small granules) and supracrestal soft tissues were conditioned by additional EMD (ie, sandwich technique[87]). *(g)* Wound closure by internal mattress sutures. *(h)* Probing at 12 months following surgery showed 7-mm CAL gain. *(i)* Radiographic view at 12 months. *(j and k)* Clinical and radiographic views 7 years following surgery. (Parts *a* to *i* reprinted with permission from Farina et al.[59])

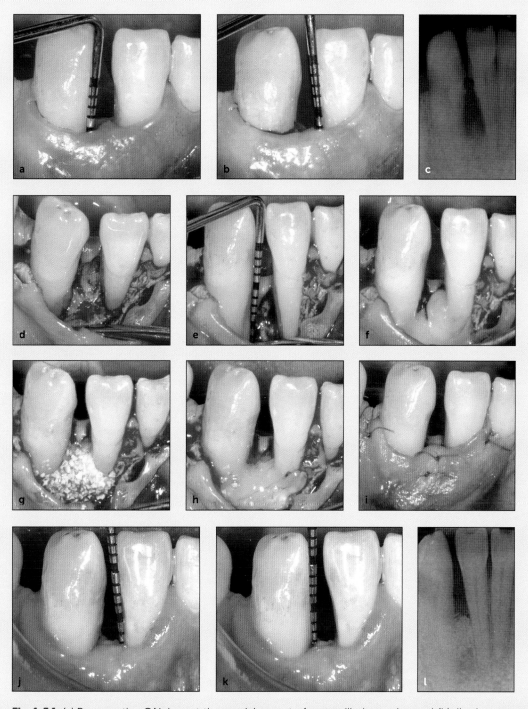

Fig 4-54 *(a)* Preoperative CAL loss at the mesial aspect of a mandibular canine and *(b)* distal aspect of a lateral incisor. *(c)* Preoperative radiographic view of the lesion. *(d)* The elevation of a buccal mucoperiosteal flap allowed for proper root/defect debridement. *(e)* Intrasurgical assessment of the intraosseous component of the defect. The defect was predominantly one-wall (lingual bony wall preserved). *(f)* According to the sandwich technique,[87] a first layer of EMD was used to condition the bone defect and the EDTA-treated root surface. *(g)* Xenograft particles (Cerabone 0.5- to 1-mm granules, Botiss-Dental) were mixed with EMD and subsequently positioned to graft the defect. *(h)* A second layer of EMD was injected to cover the grafted particles and condition the supracrestal portion of the root surface and the soft tissues. *(i)* Flap repositioning by horizontal internal mattress sutures. *(j to l)* Probing measurements and radiographic view 4 years following surgery.

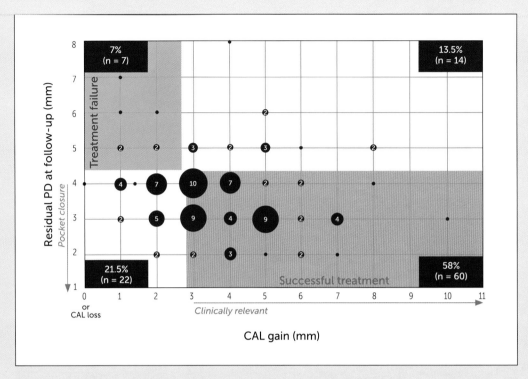

Fig 4-55 Graphic representation of CAL gain and residual PD used to define the treatment outcome of a regenerative procedure. A COM combines the "clinical relevance" of the regenerative outcome (clinically relevant if CAL gain ≥ 3 mm, clinically not relevant if CAL gain < 3 mm) as reported on the x-axis, with the "pocket closure" (closed pocket if postsurgery PD ≤ 4 mm, residual pocket if postsurgery PD > 4 mm) as reported on the y-axis. Cases falling into the *green area* are considered as successful treatments, where a clinically relevant result (6-month CAL gain ≥ 3 mm) is associated with the absence of a residual pocket (6-month residual PD ≤ 4 mm). Cases in the *red area* represent treatment failures, where a limited (≤ 3 mm) 6-month CAL gain is associated with a residual pocket (ie, 6-month PD > 4 mm).

absence of a residual pocket (ie, PD ≤ 4 mm), while treatment *failure* consists of limited (ie, ≤ 2 mm) CAL gain in association with a residual pocket. COM was used to evaluate the effect of a regenerative procedure on a cohort of patients where the intraosseous defect was accessed by SFA with and without the additional use of a regenerative device.[90] Figure 4-55 illustrates the distribution of the entire study population according to COM.[90] A successful treatment was observed in 60 patients (58%), while treatment failure was observed in 7 patients (7%). Twenty-two patients (21.5%) showed pocket closure in absence of a relevant CAL gain, while 14 patients (13.5%) had a relevant CAL gain but a residual pocket.

When different regenerative procedures are considered, differences among treatment groups are evident. For instance, a difference in patient distribution was observed between the SFA alone (SH) versus SFA with EMD + DBBM. In particular, complete success was

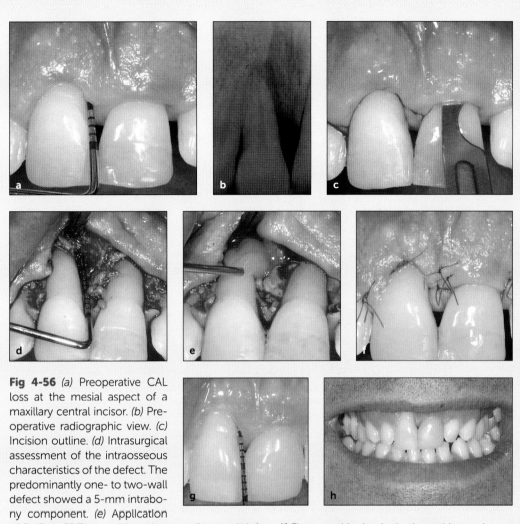

Fig 4-56 *(a)* Preoperative CAL loss at the mesial aspect of a maxillary central incisor. *(b)* Preoperative radiographic view. *(c)* Incision outline. *(d)* Intrasurgical assessment of the intraosseous characteristics of the defect. The predominantly one- to two-wall defect showed a 5-mm intrabony component. *(e)* Application of EMD to EDTA-conditioned root surface and defect. *(f)* Flap repositioning by horizontal internal mattress sutures. *(g)* Periodontal stability at 4 years following surgery. *(h)* The increase in buccal gingival recession determined an altered leveling of the gingival scalloping with consequent esthetic impairment.

obtained in 77.5% vs 48% in EMD + DBBM and SH cases, respectively. Also, treatment failure occurred less frequently in EMD + DBBM treatment (3% vs 8%, respectively).

Limiting postsurgery recession following the SFA

The stability of the buccal gingival profile may represent a treatment goal, particularly when the regenerative procedure is performed in esthetically sensitive areas of the dentition (Fig 4-56). Together with the buccal bone dehiscence, a second factor that should be considered in the development of buccal gingival recession is the gingival thickness. In this respect, previous studies have shown that thick gingival tissues exhibit a greater resistance to recession after surgical trauma and minimal tissue remodeling after various surgical procedures,

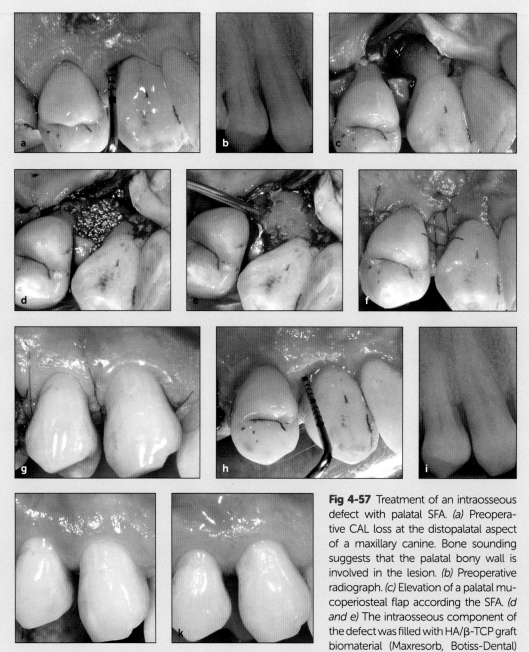

Fig 4-57 Treatment of an intraosseous defect with palatal SFA. *(a)* Preoperative CAL loss at the distopalatal aspect of a maxillary canine. Bone sounding suggests that the palatal bony wall is involved in the lesion. *(b)* Preoperative radiograph. *(c)* Elevation of a palatal mucoperiosteal flap according the SFA. *(d and e)* The intraosseous component of the defect was filled with HA/β-TCP graft biomaterial (Maxresorb, Botiss-Dental) and EMD. *(f and g)* Primary intention wound closure was obtained by the use of two internal mattress sutures and one interrupted suture. *(h and i)* Probing measurement and radiographic view at 12-month follow-up. *(j and k)* Preoperative and 12-month view of the buccal gingival profile. Note the limited postsurgery recession.

including regenerative surgery.[91,92] Thus, the presence of a deep buccal dehiscence and thin gingival tissues should be considered high-risk conditions in the development of a buccal gingival recession following surgery. To minimize this unfavorable outcome, the clinician may take advantage of the following surgical expedients:

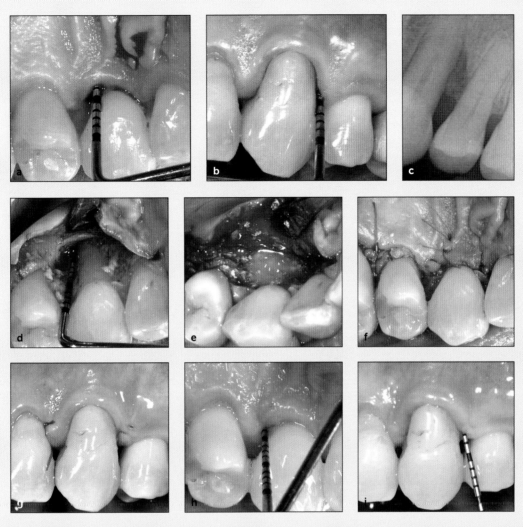

Fig 4-58 *(a and b)* Interproximal intraosseous lesion with a palatal extension at a maxillary canine. *(c)* Preoperative radiograph. *(d)* Elevation of a palatal SFA allowed for proper root/defect debridement. The intraosseous component of the defect was 7 mm deep. *(e)* A sandwich technique with EMD and HA/β-TCP graft biomaterial (Maxresorb) was used. *(f and g)* Wound closure was obtained with two internal mattress sutures. No alteration of the buccal gingival profile was evident. *(h and i)* Probing measurements at 1-year follow-up.

- The use of a palatal SFA (provided the morphology of the defect is compatible with such surgical access; Figs 4-57 and 4-58)
- The use of a connective tissue graft (CTG) or collagen membrane in addition to SFA[93] (Video 4-21, Fig 4-59)

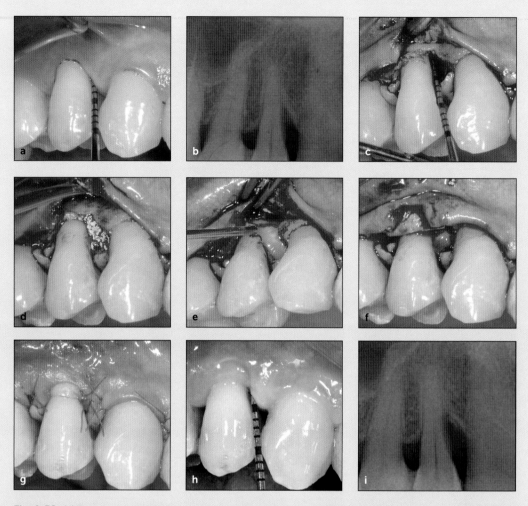

Fig 4-59 *(a)* Preoperative CAL loss at the mesial aspect of a maxillary first premolar. *(b)* Preoperative radiograph. *(c)* Intrasurgical assessment of the intraosseous characteristics of the defect. The predominantly one- to two-wall defect showed a 4-mm intrabony component. *(d and e)* The intraosseous component of the defect was treated with a combination of EMD and a bovine-derived xenograft (Cerabone 0.5- to 1-mm granules) according to the sandwich technique. *(f)* A CTG was harvested from the palate and positioned at the cementoenamel junction. *(g)* The buccal flap was repositioned and sutured, leaving the CTG partly exposed in its most coronal portion. *(h and i)* Clinical and radiographic appearance at 2 years following surgery showing the attachment gain and increased gingival dimensions.

Regarding the use of a CTG, a recent retrospective study evaluated the adjunctive effect of a CTG on the postsurgical increase in buccal gingival recession of deep intraosseous defects treated with buccal SFA in combination with EMD + DBBM.[93] After the regenerative treatment of the intrabony component of the defect with EMD + DBBM, at the operator's discretion, a CTG harvested from the palatal area was sutured at the buccal aspect of the tooth associated with the intraosseous defect. The CTG was fixed to either the flap at the level of the buccal bone dehiscence using internal mattress sutures or to the interdental papillae. The CTG was entirely covered by the buccal flap to thicken the gingival tissues or left exposed with its most coronal portion to augment the apicocoronal gingival dimension. The buccal flap was repositioned and sutured as previously described.

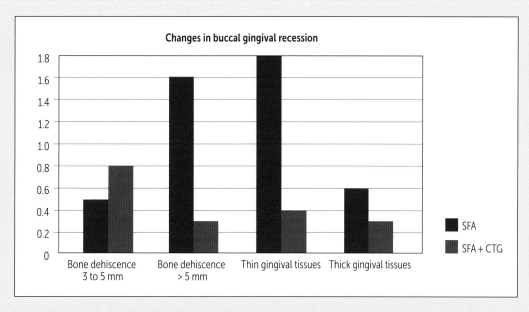

Fig 4-60 Postsurgery change in buccal gingival recession in patients treated by SFA with and without CTG according to bone dehiscence and baseline gingival thickness.

At 6 months after surgery, a trend toward better stability of the gingival profile was observed in the SFA + CTG group. In particular, in defects with a shallow (ie, 3- to 5-mm) dehiscence of the buccal bone, defects treated with SFA and SFA + CTG showed a similar 6-month increase in buccal recession of 0.8 and 0.5 mm, respectively. In defects with deep (ie, > 5-mm) buccal dehiscence, mean increase in buccal recession was pronounced (ie, 1.6 mm) in the SFA group and limited (ie, 0.3 mm) in the SFA + CTG group (Fig 4-60). When considering the 6-month changes in buccal gingival recession according to baseline gingival thickness, at sites with thin gingival tissues at baseline, the adjunctive use of a CTG significantly limited postsurgery increase in buccal recession.

Therefore, the appropriateness of the SFA + CTG procedure should be carefully evaluated in light of specific clinical indications (ie, in case of instability of the gingival margin due to severe buccal bone dehiscence and/or thin gingival tissues). In such cases, the additional use of a CTG to SFA is recommended provided the limitation in postsurgery gingival recession is of clinical relevance (see Video 4-21). A collagen matrix may be a suitable alternative to replace a CTG (Video 4-22). However, whether and to what extent this soft tissue substitute can be used to limit buccal gingival recession following SFA needs be further elucidated.

In conclusion, the adjunctive use of a CTG with the SFA seems to be indicated at defects with severe buccal bone dehiscence and/or thin gingival tissues and wherever the postsurgery gingival recession needs be prevented or limited. Figure 4-61 summarizes the decision-making process that the clinician should follow for the selection of the appropriate regenerative strategy in combination with SFA.

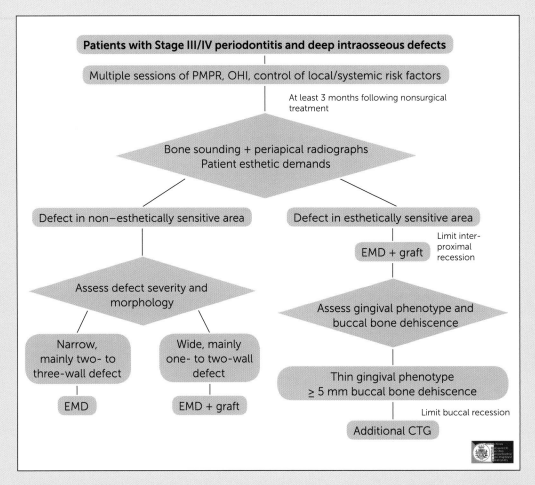

Fig 4-61 Postsurgery change in buccal gingival recession in patients treated by SFA with and without CTG according to bone dehiscence and baseline gingival thickness. PMPR, professional mechanical plaque removal; OHI, oral hygiene instruction.

REFERENCES

1. Cortellini P, Tonetti MS. Clinical concepts for regenerative therapy in intrabony defects. Periodontol 2000 2015;68:282–307.

2. Cortellini P, Tonetti MS. Focus on intrabony defects: Guided tissue regeneration. Periodontol 2000 2000;22:104–132.

3. Trombelli L, Franceschetti G, Farina R. Effect of professional mechanical plaque removal performed on a long-term, routine basis in the secondary prevention of periodontitis: A systematic review. J Clin Periodontol 2015;42(suppl 16):S221–S236.

4. Cortellini P, Pini Prato G, Tonetti MS. Periodontal regeneration of human intrabony defects with titanium reinforced membranes. A controlled clinical trial. J Periodontol 1995;66:797–803.

5. Cortellini P, Tonetti MS. Microsurgical approach to periodontal regeneration. Initial evaluation in a case cohort. J Periodontol 2001;72:559–569.

6. Ehmke B, Rüdiger SG, Hommens A, Karch H, Flemmig TF. Guided tissue regeneration using a polylactic acid barrier. J Clin Periodontol 2003;30:368–374.

7. Stavropoulos A, Mardas N, Herrero F, Karring T. Smoking affects the outcome of guided tissue regeneration with bioresorbable membranes: A retrospective analysis of intrabony defects. J Clin Periodontol 2004;31:945–950.

8. Trombelli L, Kim CK, Zimmerman GJ, Wikesjö UM. Retrospective analysis of factors related to clinical outcome of guided tissue regeneration procedures in intrabony defects. J Clin Periodontol 1997;24:366–371.

9. Trombelli L, Farina R, Minenna L, Toselli L, Simonelli A. Regenerative periodontal treatment with the single flap approach in smokers and nonsmokers. Int J Periodontics Restorative Dent 2018;38:e59–e67.

10. Tonetti M, Cortellini P, Suvan JE, et al. Generalizability of the added benefits of guided tissue regeneration in the treatment of deep intrabony defects. Evaluation in a multi-center randomized controlled clinical trial. J Periodontol 1998;69:1183–1192.

11. Steffensen B, Webert HP. Relationship between the radiographic periodontal defect angle and healing after treatment. J Periodontol 1989;60:248–254.

12. Cortellini P, Tonetti MS. Evaluation of the effect of tooth vitality on regenerative outcomes in intrabony defects. J Clin Periodontol 2001;28:672–679.

13. Cortellini P, Stalpers G, Mollo A, Tonetti MS. Periodontal regeneration versus extraction and prosthetic replacement of teeth severely compromised by attachment loss to the apex: 5-year results of an ongoing randomized clinical trial. J Clin Periodontol 2011;38:915–924.

14. Cortellini P, Tonetti MS, Lang NP, et al. The simplified papilla preservation flap in the regenerative treatment of deep intrabony defects: Clinical outcomes and postoperative morbidity. J Periodontol 2001;72:1701–1712.

15. Trejo PM, Weltman RL. Favourable periodontal regenerative outcomes from teeth with presurgical mobility: A retrospective study. J Clin Periodontol 2004;75:1532–1538.

16. Papapanou PN, Wennström JL, Gröndahl K. Periodontal status in relation to age and tooth type. A cross-sectional radiographic study. J Clin Periodontol 1988;15:469–478.

17. Ramfjord SP, Nissle RR. The modified Widman flap. J Clin Periodontol 1974;45:601–607.

18. Kirkland O. The suppurative pus pocket; its treatment by modified flap operation. J Am Dent Assoc 1931;18:1462–1470.

19. Takei HH, Han, TJ, Carranza FA Jr, Kenney EB, Lekovic V. Flap technique for periodontal bone implants. Papilla preservation technique. J Periodontol 1985;56:204–210.

20. Murphy KG. Interproximal tissue maintenance in GTR procedures: Description of a surgical technique and 1-year reentry results. Int J Periodontics Restorative Dent 1996;16:463–477.

21. Harrel SK. A minimally invasive surgical approach for periodontal regeneration: Surgical technique and observations. J Periodontol 1999;70:1547–1557.

22. Cortellini P, Prato GP, Tonetti MS. The modified papilla preservation technique. A new surgical approach for interproximal regenerative procedures. J Periodontol 1995;66:261–266.

23. Cortellini P, Prato GP, Tonetti MS. The simplified papilla preservation flap. A novel surgical approach for the management of soft tissues in regenerative procedures. Int J Periodontics Restorative Dent 1999;19:589–599.

24. Tinti C. The interproximally connected flap to treat intrabony defects: Case reports. Int J Periodontics Restorative Dent 2007;27:17–25.

25. Becker W, Becker BE, Berg L, Prichard J, Caffesse R, Rosenberg E. New attachment after treatment with root isolation procedures: Report for treated Class III and Class II furcations and vertical osseous defects. Int J Periodontics Restorative Dent 1988;8:8–23.

26. Tonetti MS, Pini-Prato G, Cortellini P. Periodontal regeneration of human intrabony defects. IV. Determinants of healing response. J Periodontol 1993;64:934–940.

27. Selvig KA, Kersten BG, Wikesjö UM. Surgical treatment of intrabony periodontal defects using expanded polytetrafluoroethylene barrier membranes: Influence of defect configuration on healing response. J Periodontol 1993;64:730–733.

28. Michaelides PL, Wilson SG. A comparison of papillary retention versus full-thickness flaps with internal mattress sutures in anterior periodontal surgery. Int J Periodontics Restorative Dent 1996;16:388–397.

29. Trombelli L, Farina R, Franceschetti G. Single flap approach in periodontal surgery [in Italian]. Dental Cadmos 2007;75:15–25.

30. Cortellini P, Pini Prato G, Tonetti MS. The modified papilla preservation technique with bioresorbable barrier membranes in the treatment of intrabony defects. Case reports. Int J Periodontics Restorative Dent 1996;16:547–559.

31. Graziani F, Gennai S, Cei S, et al. Clinical performance of access flap surgery in the treatment of the intrabony defect. A systematic review and meta-analysis of randomized clinical trials. J Clin Periodontol 2012;39:145–156.

32. Tu YK, Tugnait A, Clerehugh V. Is there a temporal trend in the reported treatment efficacy of periodontal regeneration? A meta-analysis of randomized-controlled trials. J Clin Periodontol 2008;35:139–146.

33. Trombelli L, Simonelli A, Pramstraller M, Wikesjö UM, Farina R. Single flap approach with and without guided tissue regeneration and a hydroxyapatite biomaterial in the management of intraosseous periodontal defects. J Periodontol 2010;81:1256–1263.

34. Checchi L, Montevecchi M, Checchi V, Laino G. Coronally advanced single flap in periodontal reconstructive surgery [in Italian]. Dent Cadmos 2008;76:46–58.

35. Cortellini P, Tonetti MS. Improved wound stability with a modified minimally invasive surgical technique in the regenerative treatment of isolated interdental intrabony defects. J Clin Periodontol 2009;36:157–163.

36. Zucchelli G, Mazzotti C, Tirone F, Mele M, Bellone P, Mounssif I. The connective tissue graft wall technique and enamel matrix derivative to improve root coverage and clinical attachment levels in Miller Class IV gingival recession. Int J Periodontics Restorative Dent 2014;34:601–609.

37. Trombelli L, Simonelli A, Schincaglia GP, Cucchi A, Farina R. Single-flap approach for surgical debridement of deep intraosseous defects: A randomized controlled trial. J Periodontol 2012;83:27–35.

38. Linghorne WJ, O'Connell DC. Studies in the regeneration and reattachment of supporting structures of the teeth; soft tissue reattachment. J Dent Res 1950;29:419–428.

39. Wikesjö UM, Nilvéus R. Periodontal repair in dogs: Effect of wound stabilization on healing. J Periodontol 1990;61:719–724.

40. Wikesjö UM, Nilvéus RE, Selvig KA. Significance of early wound healing on periodontal repair: A review. J Periodontol 1992;63:158–165.

41. Hiatt WH, Stallard RE, Butler ED, Badgett B. Repair following mucoperiosteal flap surgery with full gingival retention. J Periodontol 1968;39:11–16.

42. Werfully S, Areibi G, Toner M, et al. Tensile strength, histological and immunohistochemical observations of periodontal wound healing in the dog. J Periodontal Res 2002;37:366–374.

43. Yumet JA, Polson AM. Gingival wound healing in the presence of plaque-induced inflammation. J Periodontol 1985;56:107–119.

44. Cortellini P, Tonetti MS. Clinical and radiographic outcomes of the modified minimally invasive surgical technique with and without regenerative materials: A randomized-controlled trial in intrabony defects. J Clin Periodontol 2011;38:365–373.

45. Farina R, Simonelli A, Rizzi A, Pramstraller M, Cucchi A, Trombelli L. Early postoperative healing following buccal single flap approach to access intraosseous periodontal defects. Clin Oral Investig 2013;17:1573–1583.

46. Schincaglia GP, Hebert E, Farina R, Simonelli A, Trombelli L. Single versus double flap approach in periodontal regenerative treatment. J Clin Periodontol 2015;42:557–566.

47. Wachtel H, Schenk G, Böhm S, Weng D, Zuhr O, Hürzeler MB. Microsurgical access flap and enamel matrix derivative for the treatment of periodontal intrabony defects: A controlled clinical study. J Clin Periodontol 2003;30:496–504.

48. Azuma H, Kono T, Morita H, Tsumori N, Miki H, Shiomi K, Umeda M. Single flap periodontal surgery induces early fibrous tissue generation by wound stabilization [in Japanese]. J Hard Tissue Biol 2017;26:119–126.

49. Tonetti MS, Lang NP, Cortellini P, et al. Enamel matrix proteins in the regenerative therapy of deep intrabony defects. J Clin Periodontol 2002;29:317–325.

50. Cortellini P, Tonetti MS. A minimally invasive surgical technique with an enamel matrix derivative in the regenerative treatment of intra-bony defects: A novel approach to limit morbidity. J Clin Periodontol 2007;34:87–93.

51. Aimetti M, Ferrarotti F, Mariani GM, Romano F. A novel flapless approach versus minimally invasive surgery in periodontal regeneration with enamel matrix derivative proteins: A 24-month randomized controlled clinical trial. Clin Oral Invest 2017;21:327–337.

52. Vrotsos JA, Parashis AO, Theofanatos GD, Smulow JB. Prevalence and distribution of bone defects in moderate and advanced adult periodontitis. J Clin Periodontol 1999;26:44–48.

53. Tal H. The prevalence and distribution of intrabony defects in dry mandibles. J Periodontol 1984;55:149–154.

54. Zybutz M, Rapoport D, Laurell L, Persson GR. Comparisons of clinical and radiographic measurements of interproximal vertical defects before and 1 year after surgical treatments. J Clin Periodontol 2000;27:179–186.

55. Renvert S, Garrett S, Shallhorn R, Egelberg J. Healing after treatment of intraosseous defects III. Effect of osseous grafting and citric acid conditioning. J Clin Periodontol 1985;12:441–455.

56. Grimard BA, Hoidal MJ, Mills MP, Mellonig JT, Nummikoski PV, Mealey BL. Comparison of clinical, periapical radiograph, and cone-beam volume tomography measurement techniques for assessing bone level changes following regenerative periodontal therapy. J Periodontol 2009;80:48–55.

57. de Faria Vasconcelos K, Evangelista KM, Rodrigues CD, Estrela C, de Sousa TO, Silva MA. Detection of periodontal bone loss using cone beam CT and intraoral radiography. Dentomaxillofac Radiol 2012;41:64–69.

58. Walter C, Schmidt JC, Dula K, Sculean A. Cone beam computed tomography (CBCT) for diagnosis and treatment planning in periodontology: A systematic review. Quintessence Int 2016;47:25–37.

59. Farina R, Simonelli A, Minenna L, Rasperini G, Trombelli L. Single-flap approach in combination with enamel matrix derivative in the treatment of periodontal intraosseous defects. Int J Periodontics Restorative Dent 2014;34:497–506.

60. Trombelli L, Simonelli A, Minenna L, Vecchiatini R, Farina R. Simplified procedures to treat periodontal intraosseous defects in esthetic areas. Periodontol 2000 2018;77:93–110.

61. Trombelli L, Farina R, Franceschetti G, Calura G. Single-flap approach with buccal access in periodontal reconstructive procedures. J Periodontol 2009;80:353–360.

62. Nobuto T, Imai H, Suwa F, et al. Microvascular response in the periodontal ligament following mucoperiosteal flap surgery. J Periodontol 2003;74:521–528.

63. Nobuto T, Suwa F, Kono T, et al. Microvascular response in the periosteum following mucoperiosteal flap surgery in dogs: 3-dimensional observation of an angiogenic process. J Periodontol 2005;76:1339–1345.

64. Yaffe A, Fine N, Binderman I. Regional accelerated phenomenon in the mandible following mucoperiosteal flap surgery. J Periodontol 1994;65:79–83.

65. Cafffesse RG, Castelli WA, Nasjleti CE. Vascular response to modified Widman flap surgery in monkeys. J Periodontol 1981;52:1–7.

66. Crea A, Deli G, Littarru C, Lajolo C, Orgeas GV, Tatakis DN. Intrabony defects, open-flap debridement, and decortication: A randomized clinical trial. J Periodontol 2014;85:34–42.

67. Trombelli L, Heitz-Mayfield IJ, Needleman I, Moles D, Scabbia A. A systematic review of graft materials and biological agents for periodontal intraosseous defects. J Clin Periodontol 2002;29:117–135.

68. Tonetti MS, Pini-Prato G, Cortellini P. Effect of cigarette smoking on periodontal healing following GTR in infrabony defects. A preliminary retrospective study. J Clin Periodontol 1995;22:229–234.

69. Mishra A, Avula H, Pathakota KR, Avula J. Efficacy of modified minimally invasive surgical technique in the treatment of human intrabony defects with or without use of rhPDGF-BB gel: A randomized controlled trial. J Clin Periodontol 2013;40:172–179.

70. Zucchelli G, Bernardi F, Montebugnoli L, De SM. Enamel matrix proteins and guided tissue regeneration with titanium-reinforced expanded polytetrafluoroethylene membranes in the treatment of infrabony defects: A comparative controlled clinical trial. J Periodontol 2002;73:3–12.

71. Francetti L, Del Fabbro M, Basso M, Testori T, Weinstein R. Enamel matrix proteins in the treatment of intrabony defects. A prospective 24-month clinical trial. J Clin Periodontol 2004;31:52–59.

72. Liu S, Hu B, Zhang Y, Li W, Song J. Minimally invasive surgery combined with regenerative biomaterials in treating intra-bony defects: A meta-analysis. PLoS One 2016;11:e0147001.

73. Tsitoura E, Tucker R, Suvan J, Laurell L, Cortellini P, Tonetti M. Baseline radiographic defect angle of the intrabony defect as a prognostic indicator in regenerative periodontal surgery with enamel matrix derivative. J Clin Periodontol 2004;31:643–647.

74. Cortellini P, Buti J, Pini Prato G, Tonetti MS. Periodontal regeneration compared with access flap surgery in human intra-bony defects 20-year follow-up of a randomized clinical trial: Tooth retention, periodontitis recurrence and costs. J Clin Periodontol 2017;44:58–66.

75. Farina R, Simonelli A, Minenna L, et al. Change in the gingival margin profile after the single flap approach in periodontal intraosseous defects. J Periodontol 2015;86:1038–1046.

76. Nyman S, Lindhe J, Karring T, Rylander H. New attachment following surgical treatment of human periodontal disease. J Clin Periodontol 1982;9:290–296.

77. Stahl SS, Froum S, Tarnow D. Human histologic responses to guided tissue regenerative techniques in intrabony lesions. Case reports on 9 sites. J Clin Periodontol 1990;17:191–198.

78. Cortellini P, Clauser C, Prato GP. Histologic assessment of new attachment following the treatment of a human buccal recession by means of a guided tissue regeneration procedure. J Periodontol 1993;64:387–391.

79. Needleman IG, Worthington HV, Giedrys-Leeper E, Tucker RJ. Guided tissue regeneration for periodontal infra-bony defects. Cochrane Database Syst Rev 2006;19:CD001724.

80. Simonelli A, Farina R, Rizzi A, Trombelli L. Single flap approach in the reconstructive treatment of a periodontal intraosseous defect associated with a root abnormality [in Italian]. Dent Cadmos 2013;81:365–373.

81. Esposito M, Grusovin MG, Papanikolau N, Coulthard P, Worthington HV. Enamel matrix derivative (Emdogain®) for periodontal tissue regeneration in intrabony defects. Cochrane Database Syst Rev 2009;4:CD003875.

82. Sanz M, Tonetti MS, Zabalegui I, et al. Treatment of intrabony defects with enamel matrix proteins or barrier membranes: Results from a multicenter practice-based clinical trial. J Periodontol 2004;75:726–733.

83. Darby IB, Morris KH. A systematic review of the use of growth factors in human periodontal regeneration. J Periodontol 2013;84:465–476.

84. Venezia E, Goldstein M, Boyan BD, Schwartz Z. The use of enamel matrix derivative in the treatment of periodontal defects: A literature review and meta-analysis. Crit Rev Oral Biol Med 2004;15:382–402.

85. Koop R, Merheb J, Quirynen M. Periodontal regeneration with enamel matrix derivative in reconstructive periodontal therapy: A systematic review. J Periodontol 2012;83:707–720.

86. Kao RT, Nares S, Reynolds MA. Periodontal regeneration - intrabony defects: A systematic review from the AAP Regeneration Workshop. J Periodontol 2015;86(suppl 2):S77–S104.

87. Trombelli L, Annunziata M, Belardo S, Farina R, Scabbia A, Guida L. Autogenous bone graft in conjunction with enamel matrix derivative in the treatment of deep periodontal intra-osseous defects: A report of 13 consecutively treated patients. J Clin Periodontol 2006;33:69–75.

88. Froum SJ, Weinberg MA, Rosenberg E, Tarnow D. A comparative study utilizing open flap debridement with and without enamel matrix derivative in the treatment of periodontal intrabony defects: A 12-month re-entry study. J Periodontol 2001;72:25–34.

89. Listl S, Tu YK, Faggion CM Jr. A cost-effectiveness evaluation of enamel matrix derivatives alone or in conjunction with regenerative devices in the treatment of periodontal intra-osseous defects. J Clin Periodontol 2010;37:920–927.

90. Trombelli L, Farina R, Vecchiatini R, Maietti E, Simonelli A. A simplified composite outcome measure to assess the effect of periodontal regenerative treatment in intraosseous defects [epub ahead of print 22 Nov 2019]. J Periodontol doi:10.1002/JPER.190127.

91. Huang LH, Neiva RE, Wang HL. Factors affecting the outcomes of coronally advanced flap root coverage procedure. J Periodontol 2005;76:1729–1734.

92. Hwang D, Wang HL. Flap thickness as a predictor of root coverage: A systematic review. J Periodontol 2006;77:1625–1634.

93. Trombelli L, Simonelli A, Minenna L, Rasperini G, Farina R. Effect of a connective tissue graft in combination with a single flap approach in the regenerative treatment of intraosseous defects. J Periodontol 2017;88:348–356.

INDEX

Page references followed by "f" denote figures, "t" denote tables, and "b" denote boxes.

A

AAP. *See* American Academy of Periodontology.
Acellular root cementum, 19
Air polishing, 52–53, 53f
Allografts, 15
Alloplastic materials, 15
Amelogenins, 19–20
American Academy of Periodontology, 41
Amino acid glycine powder air polishing, 52
Antimicrobials, for plaque removal, 53–55, 53f–55f
Autogenous grafts, 14–15

B

Barrier membranes, 12–13
Basic fibroblast growth factor, 25
BDXs. *See* Bovine-derived xenografts.
bFGF. *See* Basic fibroblast growth factor.
Bioactive glasses, 18
Biofilm, 41, 84, 110f
Bite guard, 82, 83f
Bleeding on probing, 1, 59–60, 78
BMPs. *See* Bone morphogenetic proteins.
Bone grafts. *See also* Grafts.
    allografts, 15
    autogenous, 14–15
    in periodontal regeneration, 14–17
Bone morphogenetic proteins
    BMP-2, 26–27
    BMP-3, 27
    BMP-6, 27
    BMP-7, 27–28
    BMP-12, 28
    BMP-14, 28
    description of, 15, 26
    periodontal regeneration uses of, 26–28
    wound healing uses of, 26–28
Bone substitute, enamel matrix derivative with, 122–129, 124f, 126f–128f
BOP. *See* Bleeding on probing.
Bovine-derived xenografts, 15

C

CAL. *See* Clinical attachment level.
Calculus, 42f–43f
    Er:YAG laser removal of, 51
    manual devices for removal of, 53
    residual, after professional mechanical plaque removal, 61, 61f
    subgingival, 41f–42f, 48, 52
    supragingival, 42f, 52
Cartilage-derived morphogenetic protein 1, 27
CDMP-1. *See* Cartilage-derived morphogenetic protein 1.
Cellulose acetate laboratory filter, 12

Cemental tear, 78f
Cementum, 8, 10, 17f
Chlorhexidine gluconate, 54–55, 54f–55f
Clinical attachment level, 69f
    antimicrobial effects on, 54
    description of, 2, 13, 15
    enamel matrix derivative effects on, 120
    papilla preservation techniques' effect on, 88
    preoperative loss of, 85f
    single-flap approach effects on, 95f, 108f
Clot, fibrin, 7–9, 66–67, 111
Collagen, 7–9, 97
Collagen matrix, 10
Cone-beam computed tomography, 102
Connective tissue attachment, 8–11
Connective tissue graft with single-flap approach, 131–133, 132f–134f
Coralline xenografts, 16
Coronally positioned single-flap approach, 93
CP-SFA. *See* Coronally positioned single-flap approach.
Critical probing depth, 59

D

DBBM. *See* Demineralized bovine bone mineral.
Decalcified freeze-dried bone allografts, 15–16
Demineralized bovine bone mineral, 85f
Dental hygienist, 46
Dental plaque
    biofilm of, 41, 110f
    interdental cleaning for, 47, 47f
    interproximal cleaning for, 47
    professional mechanical plaque removal. *See* Professional mechanical plaque removal.
    self-performed control of, 46–48, 47f–48f
    tooth brushing for, 46–47, 47f
Dentin tubules, 10
DFA. *See* Double-flap approach.
DFDBA. *See* Decalcified freeze-dried bone allografts.
Diabetes mellitus, 61, 62f
Diastema, 56
Diode laser, 51
Double-flap approach
    morbidity after, 98–99
    single-flap approach versus, 93, 95f, 97–99, 97f, 99f
Doxycycline gel, 53

E

Early healing index, 95–97, 96f, 97f, 119f
EDTA. *See* Ethylenediaminetetraacetic acid.
EHI. *See* Early healing index.
Electric toothbrushes, 46
EMD. *See* Enamel matrix derivative.
Emdogain, 20–21, 22f
EMPs. *See* Enamel matrix proteins.